The
Purple World

The
Purple World

Healing the Harm in
American Health Care

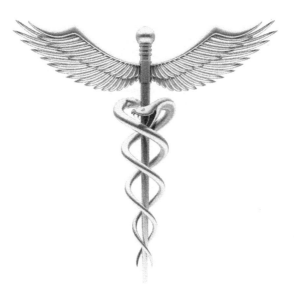

Joseph Q. Jarvis, MD, MSPH

Editorial work and production management by Eschler Editing
Cover design by Brian Halley
Interior print design and layout by Marny K. Parkin
eBook design and layout by Marny K. Parkin

Published by Scrivener Books

First Edition: May 2018
Printed in the United States of America
10 9 8 7 6 5 4 3 2 1

ISBN 978-0-9986254-8-5 (Softcover)

To my daughter Caitlin H. Jarvis,
my colleague in advocacy
for better, simpler, cheaper health care for all Americans

Contents

Acknowledgments

FOREMOST I THANK Annette W. Jarvis, my spouse, for her understanding and support of this passion of mine to heal the harm in American health care. Without Annette, none of my work on this issue leading to writing this book would have happened. I am also grateful to my children, who grew up listening to my health-policy rants and still forgive me. I am indebted to the many hundreds (thousands?) of patients through whom I have learned the practice of medicine. All doctors should humbly admit that their skill and knowledge is given as a gift to them by patients creating a debt that is never repaid. I have been blessed to work with three editors during the creation of this book. Crystal Liechty, who showed me how to give my story a meaningful shape, Kathy Jenkins, who smoothed the shape into readable prose, and Michele Preisendorf, who made that prose conform to the requirements of style. Eschler Editing and Scrivener Books, consummate professionals, for making sure this book is everything I hoped it would be and more. Leaders of the Physicians for a National Health Program (PNHP), including Cecile Rose, David Himmelstein, and Steffie Woolhandler, have taught me much of what I know about the failings of the health-insurance business model. Brent James, leader of quality improvement at Intermountain Health Care, has generously shared his insights and experience with me. The health reform proposal for Utah outlined in Chapter 11 was developed in conversation with Richard Passoth. I am deeply grateful to each of these people for their contributions to the effort that made this book possible.

Preface

ON NOVEMBER 8, 2016, the United States of America entered a purple world. What had been considered a solid blue wall in presidential politics crumbled, creating what felt like the most significant change in American governance during my lifetime. I did not vote for Mr. Trump, so I can claim no victory. Nor did I vote for Ms. Clinton, and I don't lament her loss. The American electorate became less reliably red or blue (in other words, it became more purple), and therefore much more unpredictable, more irascible, and more demanding of its government. That, I believe, is all to the good, though it is very uncertain what the electorate is demanding other than change.

A key issue in the 2016 election, a race with no real dominant policy domain, was health-care reform. That's nothing new. Americans have been attempting health-system reform for at least fifty years. More recently, the repeal of Obamacare has been the battle cry of the red side of the political aisle in every congressional election during the Obama presidency. Mr. Trump joined that chorus. And what seemed to help turn the voting world purple was the stark rise in Obamacare health-insurance premiums, an increase that was announced during the period of early voting. Mr. Trump did not articulate anything cogent about the health-care policy during the campaign that he might pursue after election, but that didn't matter: voters just knew that the health-care status quo, represented then by Ms. Clinton, was untenable. It's hard to disagree with that.

This purple-world policy vacuum creates an opportunity. Unlike President Obama, who had hammered out a policy deal with the medical industrial complex before he was even sworn in to office, Mr. Trump is apparently not going to drive health policy. And Congress, the body that should legitimately be tending the purse strings of the federal government, and therefore the national policy, has a majority that seems unlikely to agree with itself. With the Democrats in Congress simply playing Obamacare defense and the Republicans unable to articulate exactly what repeal and replace should be, American patients may find themselves without recourse when in need of health-care financing.

The Affordable Care Act, on the other hand, anticipated a rising role for state-health policy innovation beginning in 2017. During that year, the California legislature actually considered "comprehensive" health-system reform legislation (SB 562), which was touted as "single-payer reform." That bill passed the California Senate but was held up in the California Assembly, where ultimately a select committee issued a report rejecting it. "Single-payer health reform" refers to a proposed change in health policy in the United States. The current status has multiple payers for health care, both public (Medicare, Medicaid, CHIP, VA, Indian Health Service, etc.) and private (usually for-profit health insurance, but also HMOs, and BC/BS, which can be nonprofit). Single-payer health-system reform proposes to replace these multiple payers for health care with one, single paying entity in a given region (such as a state) or throughout the entire nation ("Medicare for All"). The state-health policy innovation made possible by the Affordable Care Act does not explicitly call for single-payer health-system reform, but it does not exclude it either. However, if a state, such as California, were to decide through legislation or ballot initiative to attempt single-payer health-system reform, an act of Congress enabling that reform would be essential. Likewise, single-payer health-system reform on the national level ("Medicare for All") would require an act of Congress. Maybe this brave new purple world will finally offer a Tenth Amendment opportunity in health policy. That is what this book proposes.

I didn't write it in the weeks after the election. It has been several decades since I began studying medicine and lived through the experiences I tell about in this book. Back then I had a native belief in the American way of government, which I had been taught was to be of, by, and for the people. But along the way I began to doubt.

I had patients in my family practice in the 1980s who simply could not afford the simplest prescription for a child's earache. I know from observation that poor medical care can put even middle-income families outside the realm of American prosperity and leave them there for multiple generations. Despite what donated medicines and other resources I could cobble together for these families, they were hurting, and I could not do much about it. The Sisters of the Holy Cross, who made hospital care possible for my patients, did so at the cost of a burgeoning debt. Eventually they had to sell their hospital to a for-profit business, which removed any options in Salt Lake City for what was called "indigent" care. Government of, by, and for the people could not seem to provide care to many of its people, but government health programs seemed very able to make the medical industrial complex very profitable. The wonders of modern medicine and public health, which had been made possible largely through the combined efforts of all the people, were denied to millions, most of whom had paid the world's highest tax rates to support clinical science and health-care delivery.

By the time the nuns sold their hospital in Salt Lake City, I had moved on in search of a public-health career that would make a difference. The early chapters of this book are about that search. After working in federal and state government and practicing medicine in academic medical centers in Colorado, Nevada, and the District of Columbia, I returned to Salt Lake City with serious doubts about whether American government at any level could really help American families with health-care problems. I did everything I could think of to draw attention to the plight of American patients who were overcharged while they were being both over- and under-cared for: I published op-ed pieces in most major Utah newspapers, did radio and TV interviews, lobbied the legislature, started a nonprofit health-policy advocacy group, ran for office twice, gave hundreds of speeches, attended political conventions and rallies, and helped on campaigns. But nothing changed. So I decided to write this book. I titled it *The Purple World* because I hope to persuade people to vote as unpredictable, irascible, purple-change agents rather than dyed-in-the-wool red and blue partisans.

And then November 8, 2016, happened. And the Purple World emerged.

Chapter One

What's Golden in Medicine?

WAS BORN DURING the so-called "Golden Age" of medicine. Well, at least some people thought it was golden. I'm not a medical historian, nor is this a book about the history of my profession, but it's useful for people interested in "modern" medicine to contemplate how Western civilization came upon this vast and very expensive enterprise. And how it became so much more vast and expensive in the United States than anywhere else in the world. Nearly 20 percent of our American gross domestic product is spent on health care, while the average first-world country elsewhere in the world devotes about half that much economic productivity to health care. And they're all measurably in better health than Americans. We're spending about $3 trillion each year, about $1 trillion more than the rate spent by other wealthy nations, without anything to show for it.[1]

Many Americans have come to believe that we have the best health-care system in the world. Americans have a tendency to see themselves as the best in everything, so perhaps our assertion, self-serving as it is, simply belies our native jingoism. But no one, American or otherwise, can pretend that Americans invented modern medical science. That clearly happened in Europe, sometimes intentionally, other times serendipitously.

One biographer, Wendy Moore, asserted that a Scot, John Hunter, living in eighteenth-century London, invented the clinical science of surgery. At the age of twenty, he went to London to apprentice with his older brother, William, in his growing enterprise—an anatomy school.

Would-be surgeons from around the British Empire were increasingly desirous to gain expertise in dissection, a skill set they could learn only from a teacher practiced in the craft who had access to cadavers.

John proved to be adept at both acquiring dead bodies and carving them up. His reputation as a body snatcher disgusted and intrigued the London populace, but his skill as a surgeon was even more widely acclaimed—he even attended the royal family. This combination of the sinister and the salubrious was said to have made John Hunter the model for Robert Louis Stevenson's *Strange Case of Dr. Jekyll and Mr. Hyde*, published approximately a century after Hunter's death.[2]

After becoming an expert anatomist, John Hunter launched himself into a surgical career, but with a difference. Rather than accept the then traditional methods of surgery, he insisted on observing his patients for evidence of what actually worked and then altering his practices of care to match what methods made for best patient outcomes. For example, during a tour of duty as an army surgeon during the Seven Years War (known as the French and Indian War in the American colonies), Hunter took advantage of a chance incident involving five captured French soldiers to make observations about war-wound healing. Each of these soldiers had sustained a wound during battle. Unable to retreat with their regiment as the British advanced, they hid out in an abandoned farmhouse for four days before being discovered. Because they were in hiding, no surgeon had operated on their wounds. Surgical tradition of the time required that bullet wounds be explored and enlarged. In the era prior to the discovery of antiseptic technique and long before antibiotics, infection was the universal result of probing war wounds, leading to catastrophic suppuration, sepsis, and death.

Hunter noted that the five French soldiers actually were healing better than if they'd been probed by a surgeon, and eventually healed completely—including the French soldier with a through-and-through chest wound. Thereafter, Hunter limited his wound exploration on the battlefield to those cases where bleeding was excessive or bone fragments were found. Generally, he did as little as possible and let nature do the healing.

The results overcame the doubts of his detractors, who were clinging to the dictums of ancient practices like bloodletting.

In an era when bloodletting was considered a cure for everything from colds to smallpox, surgeon John Hunter was a medical innovator, an eccentric, and the person to whom anyone who has ever had surgery probably owes his or her life. A review of Moore's biography of John Hunter printed in the *New England Journal of Medicine* agrees with Moore's subtitle assessment of Dr. Hunter, stating, "John Hunter is rightly regarded as the founder of scientific surgery." He died an old man after a long and successful career.[3]

Not so for Ignaz Semmelweis, the Austro-Hungarian obstetrician who first conducted observations that eventually made antiseptic practices common in medical care. Dr. Semmelweis took his medical training in Vienna and, after graduation in 1847, became an assistant to the chief professor of obstetrics at the Vienna General Hospital. There were two obstetrical services in the hospital: the first clinic was run by the physicians and had a maternal mortality rate of 10 percent due to puerperal fever (childbed fever), while the second clinic was run by midwives and had less than half that rate of maternal mortality. The difference in death rates was well-known, and women in labor literally begged to be admitted to the second clinic.

Dr. Semmelweis took the death toll of patients in his service personally. (One can only wish same were true of American doctors. American patients would be well served if our doctors paid close attention to the medical errors in hospitals that make preventable patient injury the fifth leading cause of death in our country. For instance, nearly half of all surgeries involve some kind of medication error or unintended drug side effect).

He began to consider how the care in the first clinic differed from that delivered in the second. In doing so, he was taking on then traditional and long-held views of medicine concerning the origin of disease, namely that imbalances in the patient's four humors accounted for illness. Prior to the Semmelweis's study of the different rates of disease between the two different obstetrical clinics, no one had considered the possibility that factors external to the patient might actually be causing disease. It was universally thought that patients got sick because there was something wrong with the patients.

The breakthrough for Dr. Semmelweis came when he noted that the postmortem findings of his good friend and fellow doctor, who died from an infection after he was accidently stabbed by a scalpel during an autopsy, were identical to those of patients who died from childbed fever.

He therefore postulated that something contagious existed in cadaverous materials and, noting that physicians—but not midwives—performed autopsies, believed he'd found the reason for the higher rate of childbed fever in the first clinic. As chief resident, he instituted a policy of handwashing with chlorinated lime before attending any living patients, and the rate of childbed fever in the first clinic dropped to zero, making Dr. Semmelweis the first practitioner of continuous quality improvement in health care.

However, his findings were not accepted by the Viennese medical establishment, and he was forced to resign his position and return to Hungary, his native land. There, he grew increasingly despondent about his failure to persuade physicians to wash their hands and was eventually placed in an asylum, where he died, ironically, of sepsis in 1865. (It should drive all of us crazy that we still have trouble persuading doctors to wash their hands often enough.) One of my infectious-disease professors in medical school, trying to emphasize the ubiquitous nature of microbial risk, once said that if urine were red and stool were blue, we would live in a purple world. That world is especially purple in hospitals, the place where infections—particularly those that are hard to treat—are most common in American communities.

Ultimately, Dr. Semmelweis's ideas about handwashing gained acceptance in France and England, and then scientific credibility as first Dr. Pasteur in France and then Dr. Lister in England, elaborated on the germ theory of disease. Antiseptic technique revolutionized the care of patients and, for the first time, made it possible that the care of a physician was more likely to help than harm the patient.

By World War I, physicians were impressed enough with antiseptics that they began treating war wounds with the direct application of various antibacterial chemicals. Nonetheless, as observed by Captain Alexander Fleming, another Scotsman who'd received medical training in London, infected wounds were killing soldiers constantly. Dr. Fleming surmised that the antiseptic chemicals themselves were doing more harm than good. He documented that many disease-causing bacteria were hidden deep within wounds and not affected by the surface application of antiseptics.

His findings were ignored by his colleagues, who went about practicing medicine as they'd been taught without recognizing the harm they were doing. Most doctors practicing today in America are too busy to look at how their methods may be harming patients. By which I mean that they're too distracted by the way we do health-care business in the United States. During my last stint as a clinician actually taking care of patients, I found I was required to spend as much time dealing with insurance-claims agents as I did actually caring for patients.

After the war, Fleming returned to his research on bacteriology in London, where he serendipitously discovered the antibiotic penicillin about a decade after the armistice. It took another decade for others (not Fleming) to figure out how to mass produce and use penicillin. By D-Day near the end of World War II, however, all of the wounded in the Allied forces enjoyed the advantage over infection provided by penicillin. Dr. Fleming never profited from his discovery beyond receiving the Nobel Prize for Medicine in 1945. In fact, there's no evidence he ever thought he should profit from it. Not to say that being a doctor shouldn't provide a good living. All health professionals work hard and have difficult tasks and should be rewarded commensurately. As should those who own a business that participates meaningfully in the care of patients, such as a pharmaceutical firm. But pursuit of profit in health care now far outsizes the traditional motivation to find a way to help reduce the suffering caused by illness and injury.

Penicillin is probably the most important discovery of the past one thousand years. Its discovery epitomizes everything great about the development of modern medical science. Those whose focus on the history of medicine is principally on clinical science often call the first half of the twentieth century, ending about when I was born, the golden era of medicine. During that relatively short span of time, the efforts of dozens of European clinical scientists, like Hunter and Semmelweis, came to fruition. The basic medical sciences of anatomy and physiology yielded information that allowed physicians to escape the superstitions of the past, including bloodletting to alter body humors.

Suddenly, it seemed, it was possible to get an accurate diagnosis concerning what really was ailing the patient. And treatments, at first mostly surgical, but eventually, and still increasingly, often pharmacological, became effective. Naturally, patients (meaning all of us at one time or another) wanted in on this.

Each of us can be grateful to Fleming for realizing the importance of his chance observations in a bacteriology laboratory. However, the clamor for penicillin and other wonder drugs created the modern business of pharmacotherapy, a vast money-making enterprise. And the clamor for surgery increased demand for hospital beds and doctors. Meeting these demands for medical care created business opportunities, something far more interesting to Americans than clinical science.

Not to say that Americans hadn't taken any notice of the medical breakthroughs in Europe. One of Dr. John Hunter's premier students was an American from Philadelphia, Philip SyngPhysick (great name for a doctor), who later became professor of surgery at the University of Pennsylvania and taught his pupils to follow the Hunter methods of observation and deduction. US government funds helped to develop mass-production methods for penicillin. And with the Flexner report published in 1915, American medical schools more quickly adapted to the educational demands of reliably and uniformly training physicians in the newly robust clinical sciences. But American ingenuity really thrilled to the business possibilities of clinical science, leading to a different slant on the golden era of medicine.

With better treatments available in the early decades of the twentieth century, it became increasingly useful to receive medical care in a hospital, and as physicians became better and more uniformly trained and prepared to help patients, Americans became increasingly interested in getting hospital and physician care. Paying for these new services, however, was a challenge for many patients. The barter system where the local doc received farm produce as his fee rapidly became obsolete. More importantly, hospitals wanted more "customers" and for them to be able to pay for their care. Enter the enterprising American knack for business.

The first real health-insurance plan was invented in Texas during the Depression. About 1,500 teachers agreed to pay in advance (the first health-insurance premium) for up to twenty-one days of hospitalization per year. This became the first Blue Cross plan. At about the same time, Blue Shield plans also evolved as a means to pay for physician services. Originally, these plans were "community rated," meaning that all members of the plan paid the same premium. By 1940, about 10 percent of the American workforce had an employment-based health benefit. What happened next is an illustration of the law of unintended consequences.

While the American and British governments were spending money to develop the mass production of penicillin for the war effort, American manufacturers of weapons and all other things required to supply the Allied military were having difficulty getting and keeping a sufficiently large labor force. The men were in uniform, so the women were needed in the factories and yards. But the 1942 Stabilization Act, in an attempt to control inflation, ruled out raising wages to attract workers. Health benefits, however, were allowed and even encouraged under the act due to the fact that they weren't counted as income to the employees and therefore went untaxed. This law, which was not rescinded at the end of the war, in effect made the employer the favored source of health financing in the United States because of the unintended consequence of an act of Congress meant to help with the war effort.

The government subsidy of employment-based health benefits through exempting those benefits from taxation grew to be about half a trillion dollars a year, present day. And Americans eagerly claimed the tax-free goodies—by 1950, over half of the nation had employment-based health insurance. Health insurers, like all corporate health enterprises, love to talk about free markets and talk down "socialized medicine." But I guarantee you, if the government-sheltered tax advantages of employment-based health benefits had never existed, or had been eliminated at the end of World War II, the United States would never have become the haven for so-called "private" health insurance. Because these benefits are heavily subsidized by tax credits, those who sell them have no business decrying other publicly funded health programs as "socialism."

Propped up by the federal government as they were, health insurers went about their business making money with a vengeance. They quickly realized that some people made more claims for health care than others. So they invented experience rating (charging premiums based upon how many claims had been filed in previous years) and did away with community rating (where everyone was charged the same premium no matter how much health care they needed). Insurers competed with each other to get the business of the healthiest populations and avoided insuring those likely to be ill or injured. Preexisting conditions, even if relatively benign, like acne, became grounds for refusal to offer a health-insurance policy. Naturally, those with previous ailments (who, for instance, might've been unable to work because of illness) and those who might be older, were soon left behind by the burgeoning insurance industry. You can't make money selling health insurance to the old and sick. Thus, by the 1960s, there was a need for Medicare (government-based health insurance for the elderly) and Medicaid (government-based health insurance for the poor, who were often sick).

American taxpayers have always been generous (in a bipartisan fashion) when it comes to paying for health services. We pay taxes to build hospitals, train doctors and nurses, fund medical research, and provide community clinics. We do this not because anyone has a constitutional right to health care but because we Americans know that health care is part of the infrastructure that makes the American dream possible. Likewise, Americans recognize the economic value of building roads and highways connecting our cities and towns across the country. No one has a constitutional right to asphalt, but nonetheless, I can drive from my house to the White House without impediment, and no one calls that the socialized highway system. We realize that no one citizen can actually afford to build the necessary roads, so we build them together. Likewise, American taxpayers have always realized that no patient can actually pay the real cost of providing necessary health care, so we make arrangements to fund it together.

I once had a conversation with a retired health-insurance executive who worked during the post–World War II era as health insurance "products" were first evolving. He was so proud of what had been accomplished; how he and others had figured out the best techniques for extracting profit from the health-insurance revenue stream, never mentioning or probably even understanding how dependent that stream is on our tax dollars.

What is so clear from even a cursory observation of the business practices of American health insurers is that not only do they charge higher premiums to those with health-care problems, sometimes they make the premiums so punitive that those "sick" people won't (or can't) buy their product at all. Or they only agree to sell insurance to someone who can walk up the several flights of stairs to the only office where health insurance policy applications are accepted, conveniently located in a walk-up high-rise building. The application process is intentionally increasingly complex, only partly so that the underwriter (the person responsible for rating the applicant's health experience) can determine what premium to charge. With a complex application, chances are good that the applicant will make an error. And errors, even trivial ones, can be used later if that applicant becomes a beneficiary with a major and costly health-care problem. Health insurers routinely scour the applications of sick beneficiaries, find an error, and then claim bad faith by the applicant and rescind their health-insurance policy after the fact.

Or the health insurer can (and routinely does) write a policy such that it has unilateral control over changing health benefits, leaving a loophole allowing that insurer to deny a claim because the policy no longer covers a needed service. Sometimes health insurers won't agree to contractual terms with doctors or hospitals specializing in the care of expensive diseases, then fail to provide notice to their beneficiaries. Some health insurers will start the review of all claims by simply denying them and hoping (usually successfully) that many beneficiaries will go ahead and pay for the health care themselves. I have experienced this claims-denial tactic personally when, after my son spent an hour in an emergency room with a nosebleed I spent ten hours dealing with the health insurer to get the claim paid. Yes, health-insurance executives are a tricky bunch. And these tricks are expensive. Overhead in the US health-insurance industry runs routinely above 20 percent of premium. But from the insurer's perspective, denying applications and denying claims will grow profits, no matter what it costs. And no matter what it does to sick and injured people.

Initially, doctors fought the formation of health-insurance plans just like they fought the New Deal proposal for national health insurance. The American Medical Association was able to defeat the Roosevelt administration during the Depression, but the growth of employment-based health benefits during World War II was unstoppable because it had the big health business lobby behind it, the same lobby that later wrote the bill creating Obamacare and which is still influencing Congress as it considers Trumpcare (or is it Ryancare?). After the war, as more patients came to doctors with insurance, physicians enjoyed remarkable growth in income. In fact, I've been told that doctors back then could decide what amenities they wanted (luxury cars, country-club memberships, travel, etc.) and then arrange their fees to provide themselves with the income needed to fill those longings. Revenues were better for hospitals as well. So-called "billed charges" (what hospitals billed for goods and services provided) have taken on a surreal (very purple world) quality, with aspirin tablets showing up on hospital patient invoices costing several dollars. Even the toilet paper cost will bankrupt you. People who focus on the business of medicine (as opposed to the clinical science) often refer to the decades immediately after World War II as the golden era of medicine, when health care first began to make doctors wealthy. As a card-carrying member of the baby-boom generation, I was born right in the middle of this era. I confess, the wealth of the doctors I knew as a child was part of the attraction I felt to the profession of medicine. I wasn't alone. When I applied to medical school in the late 1970s, I was told there were ten applications for every freshman medical student placed across the country. I applied to ten schools and was granted interviews by only two. Only one of those offered me admission, initially on a waiting list. I felt very lucky to have gained admission to the University of Utah School of Medicine in 1978.

As I began my medical studies, employment-based health insurance covered virtually all working Americans and their dependents. But the cost of health care began making employers think differently about the wisdom of purchasing health insurance, even with the federal tax code exempting the benefit from income and payroll taxes. By the time President Barack Obama took office, only two-thirds of American workers and their dependents still had a health benefit. And the creativity of health-insurance executives had shifted many of the costs of care to the patients and away from the employers and insurers. Trumpcare, at least as proposed, would further push the costs of care onto individual patients and their families.

Copayments, deductibles, coinsurance, and point-of-service payments are all examples of the methods now deployed to force the insured to pay more for care. Health insurance no longer protects the beneficiary from financial disaster in the event of major illness or injury. The most common cause of personal bankruptcy in the United States is the cost of health care, and most of those going bankrupt due to illness or injury were insured at the time their health problems started. In no other first-world country will you find bake sales to raise money for cancer chemotherapy; only in the USA. (As this book was being written, a notice appeared in the *Chicago Tribune* online edition about how the students at a private school in the Windy City held a Go Purple fundraiser for their coach, who has pancreatic cancer.)

Health insurance is the most expensive, wasteful, inefficient, and useless way to pay for health care ever invented. It would long ago have been thrown on the scrap heap of American history if not for the fact that the American government at all levels—federal, state, and local—has consistently propped up this lousy business model. And the biggest propping up of health insurance is the Affordable Care Act, or Obamacare, which requires the populace to buy this wasteful product or pay a financial penalty. The health-insurance industry, who wrote the bill, of course, is happy with Obamacare. But in what world, other than the purple world of American health policy, is the mandated buying and selling of a product called a free market?

I didn't learn anything about health insurance or the business of American health care in medical school. The entire focus of my training was on the clinical science. In retrospect, what I can say about my training was that, despite all of the marvels of modern medicine, my professors oversold what clinical science can do. During orientation just before my first semester as a medical student began, for instance, a professor stood at the front of my class and told us that there is no death that is not caused by disease, no disease that cannot be better studied and understood, and once understood, no illness that cannot not be eventually treated and overcome. Even then I had my doubts. After his speech, we commenced an intense year of studying all the essential sciences of modern medicine: anatomy, physiology, histology, biochemistry, pharmacology, with the basics of physical examination and patient history thrown in. Every professor would begin his one-hour lecture by dimming the lights and turning on a slide projector. Eight hours later, at the end of the lecture day, we'd have five hundred to seven hundred pages of reading assigned. Every two weeks or so we would have examinations. The best I could do was memorize and cram, then forget everything so I could take in and regurgitate the next two weeks' worth of material. Every so often a professor would throw in that half of what we were learning was likely to be wrong and that those errors would be made obvious as future clinical science was published.

The second year of my medical training consisted principally of a series of units called organ systems. The principle professors for each organ system were clinical scientists: dermatologists for the skin, cardiologists for the circulatory system, etc. They reviewed the basic anatomy and physiology of the organ they knew best and then began to review the principle types of pathologies (things that can go wrong) that could occur within their specialty. Pathologists tend to be dry lecturers. We also received lectures on the pharmacology (the science of how medications work) of the common treatments for each organ system. Pharmacologists, at least at the University of Utah, were better speakers. But the didactic, dull nature of dimmed rooms, viewing a new slide each minute, hours upon hours each day, still sapped the energy from me without permanently enlightening me, or so it felt. And I encountered professors who seemed to doubt whether I could ever become a good clinician. It was small comfort that my classmates were likewise receiving rough treatment.

Those were two very hard years of my life, epitomized by the two weeks for final examinations at the end of my first semester. These two weeks happened to coincide exactly with my wife's final examinations in law school. We had an eight-month-old baby boy who spent those two weeks with a painful ear infection, requiring one of us to attend to him constantly. As it happened, we each had exams every other day, and my off day was her day to take an exam. So for two weeks we traded off studying for twenty-four hours, usually at school overnight, and then returning home after the exam to take care of the sick baby while the other one left to study. I don't know how we did it.

As I continued into the years of clinical training, which included the third and fourth years of medical school and three years of family-practice residency, I hoped for a more interesting learning experience. And I found that actually attending the sick and injured was fascinating. With time, I began to feel more comfortable in my role as care provider, though clinical learning came at a cost of days and nights on call. As an intern, I was training in the hospital where, just recently, the first artificial heart had been implanted: the Jarvik heart, named after its inventor.

My patients routinely mistook my name, Jarvis, for his. And for a while, I received a lot of undeserved deference from my patients, until

I learned to disclose at the outset of each encounter that I was Dr. Jarvis, not Dr. Jarvik. I also had to learn the harsh reality of exposure to microbiological agents. As a third-year medical student during a winter rotation in a children's hospital, I became ill with a respiratory virus causing children to require hospitalization. My then two-year-old son was in turn made ill through contact with me (the purple world strikes again) and was hospitalized and near death for seventy-two hours. His medical care would have bankrupted us, even though by then my wife was a federal employee with health insurance, but for the fact that the doctors and hospitals extended professional courtesy to me and did not require payment of the coinsurance.

But undeserved deference is the stuff of modern medicine. Modern hospitals and doctors have earned the reputation for immense capability in the face of disease by overcoming the common infectious killers of bygone eras: pneumonia, plague, consumption, and venereal disease. Throw in some acute surgical conditions, like appendicitis and bowel obstruction, and one can comprehend the impact of modern medicine. Average life span in the United States at the beginning of the twentieth century was about forty to fifty years. By the turn of the millennium a century later, those averages had nearly doubled. And medicine seemed to take all the credit.

But what I saw at the bedside was definitely not that story. The gains on infectious diseases seemed to be giving way. Viral ailments were not responding to pharmacotherapy. Bacterial agents were mutating and becoming impervious to penicillin and other antibiotics. New infectious diseases were arising, like AIDS, which were not treatable. Chronic diseases of the heart, lungs, liver, and neurological system were not improving despite the many therapies we were taught to apply. I believe the five-year survival of heart-failure patients, at least at the time I was in training, had hardly improved with the application of modern medicine. It seemed to me I was about to enter a profession in which I would know many things, but few of the facts would have much impact. That is, until I had some experience in obstetrics and in pediatrics.

Maternal mortality (death during pregnancy, labor, or delivery) was 5 percent for each pregnancy and 20 percent for a reproductive lifetime in the United States at the turn of the nineteenth to the twentieth century. That means that one in twenty pregnancies ended with the death of the mother, and one in five women died during their years of fertility of causes related to pregnancy and delivery. These facts by themselves accounted for much of the sentiment leading to the creation of Mother's Day (a movement led by a woman surnamed Jarvis, who is no relation to me). Beginning with Semmelweis, but really accelerating in the twentieth century with the application of surgical and antiseptic techniques, maternal mortality had precipitously fallen.

Over the years I practiced family medicine, including obstetrics, I had no patients of my own who died in pregnancy, labor, or childbirth. I knew of less than a handful while serving as a resident on obstetrical services in various hospitals. Virtually all of these pregnancies produced babies with vigorous health, only a few of whom would become ill during childhood. Because of the advent of childhood vaccines for mumps, measles, rubella, polio, tetanus, hepatitis, chicken pox, and a growing list of other diseases, childhood illnesses became rarer. Of course, I saw cases of severe illness and death at the children's hospital, mostly due to congenital causes, cancer, or trauma. But even the sickest child seemed to have enormous physiological reserves. Recovery seemed more likely on a pediatric ward.

I briefly considered entering into psychiatric training. During the third year of medical school, every student was required to spend six weeks on the acute psychiatric ward. I found myself engaged by the manifestations of psychotic disorders and, even as a medical student, felt like I could contribute to the care of these patients. My principal duty at the psychiatric ward was to conduct a comprehensive clinical history and physical examination on patients admitted during my days on-call and be sure that this information was available in the patient chart.

I would also work with the on-call resident to be sure that the proper orders were written for each patient. On one occasion, while interviewing a very large man—more than four hundred pounds—who was being admitted with psychotic problems and a tendency to violence, I was carefully reviewing all possible organ system problems (a tedious part of the patient history) and asked him if he had any symptoms related to gastrointestinal disease.

He responded that, yes, he did have gastrointestinal symptoms. He went on to say that his GI problem was hunger pains and, further, that if I did not get him a hot dog and a milkshake, he would pick me up and throw me through the window of the room where we were sitting. I went out to the nurses' station, picked up his chart, and wrote an order for hot dogs and milkshakes as needed for anxiety, which the on-call psychiatry resident countersigned. We were able to finish the intake interview without further incident.

Not so with another man admitted during my psychiatry rotation. He was a young adult who unfortunately had the first psychotic break associated with schizophrenia one afternoon while riding on the bus. He began hearing voices that terrified him. So he found the most remote space at the back of the bus and hid there. As the bus driver was finishing his shift and preparing to drive back to the maintenance yard, he asked the young man to leave the bus. The response was incoherent and violent. The bus driver called the police. Several officers tried to remove the young man from the bus but found they could not bring enough force to bear on him in the corner he was squeezed into. So they had the bus driver take the bus to the hospital emergency room.

There, with the help of an injection administered on the bus, he was restrained and taken to the psych ward. I made an attempt to collect the necessary information but found the patient too disturbed and left most of the job to be done the next morning. He'd calmed down overnight and had been let out of his restraints. He and I completed his medical history and physical examination, but as we did so, he became increasingly anxious and upset. He fixated on my name tag, pointing to it and reading my name repeatedly. I responded by pointing to his name, which was posted on the door of his hospital room, and helping him read that. Then we looked up our names in the phone book and read them again. We repeated this activity over and over as he became increasingly agitated. At midday, a nurse came into his room with his lunch, and I excused myself to take a break in the cafeteria.

While there, I received an urgent overhead page (the only time in my medical school career) to return to the psych ward. My patient had gone to the bathroom and would not come out. He was back in his full psychotic state from the evening before. The room was too small for staff to enter and restrain him. I was given the job of talking him out of the lavatory and into his restraints. I tried having him focus on my name tag and repeat my name, which he attempted. That's when I discovered he'd defecated while on the toilet and had scooped up the feces and placed it in his mouth. He sprayed me with feces every time he tried to speak (a real purple-world experience). I stuck with the task, however, and eventually got him just outside the door, where he was restrained by the staff and injected with medication.

The attending physician to whom I reported as a medical student told me I deserved the afternoon off and sent me home. I think he was mindful of the pitiful state of my clothes. My wife also found my clothes to be offensive when I arrived home. She instructed me to strip in the backyard so she could hose me down before admitting me to the house. The clothes were tossed in the trash barrel outside.

That was perhaps my most memorable moment as a medical student. I was energized by the experience, but my wife found nothing worthy of interest. When I told her I was considering the possibility of entering the psychiatric field, she bluntly told me she found that intolerable. She never wanted to hear of anything like that defecating patient again.

Psychiatry and behavioral health are the poor stepchildren of medicine. Mental illness, while deserving the attention of clinical science, is difficult for the average person to explain or experience. Many people find the behavior of mentally ill or addicted people to be repulsive and intrusive. Some wonder why they don't simply stop these unwanted behaviors or feelings. I actually did have a patient on the psychiatric ward who, though admitted with a diagnosis of schizophrenia, admitted that he knew how to fake the condition and did so in order to avail himself of warm quarters and food during cold weather.

Another man, who did not assert that he was faking schizophrenia, gained admission to the psych ward by throwing a rock into the window of a fire station. He knew he needed help but didn't know how to ask for it. Of course, many times, the behaviors of people with mental illness, and especially addictions, can be dangerous to other people. All of these observations have tended to push society toward handling these problems through law enforcement, the courts, and jail, rather than with a robust public health-system response. I would've enjoyed a career with those kinds of challenges, I think. But my wife's preferences mattered to me, so I turned elsewhere.

I learned in obstetrics and pediatrics the value of public health and preventive medicine. Most of the improvement in the health of human populations had occurred prior to the application of clinical science to the bedside. Improved sanitation, nutrition, housing, and work conditions had transformed maternity and childhood from hazardous to wholesome. This was why I chose public health as my career. Obstetricians make many times the salary given public-health physicians. Indeed, 99 percent of funds spent on health in the United States are spent on clinical care. Only 1 percent is spent on public-health measures. Yet most of our community health achievements are made in the public-health sector.

I wanted to be in on that achievement.

Chapter Two

Exploiting Pathology for Profit

OR MANY READERS, public health probably sounds like government, and government sounds like bureaucracy. We've been told repeatedly that government is the problem and can't be the solution, or something to that effect. We all know bureaucracy is a daily reality, especially for government workers. But the sheer lunacy of what unfettered bureaucracy leads to can be downright dangerous, especially when unchecked. What does it mean for citizens when government employees, who's first loyalty lies with protecting their jobs, are in charge of making important health decisions for the nation? But bureaucracy exists in the private sector as well. So, alternatively, what does it mean for patients when health-insurance employees are in charge of making important health decisions while having the profit of their employer as the first priority?

My first year out of medical training (1986–87), I worked as a medical officer in the Office of Occupational Medicine, Directorate of Technical Support, Occupational Safety and Health Administration (OSHA) in the US Department of Labor in Washington, DC.

It was during the part of the Reagan administration when Nancy Reagan started the "Just Say No" to drugs campaign. In August—a month or so after I started what was intended to be a one-year postgraduate federal public-health experience—I received a memorandum from what the civil servants in the agency (career bureaucrats) called the "Republican" floor, authored by a deputy assistant secretary (probably some hotshot political wonk whose appointment was a reward for working on the Reagan campaign) who asked that I provide her with a definitive proposal for enforcing drug testing in American workplaces by close of business that afternoon.

That started a frenzied, one-week chain of events I began by attempting to explain to the deputy assistant secretary why OSHA could not simply or easily pass rules requiring nationwide, universal employee drug testing. I'd had very little experience with drug testing in the workplace but had become acquainted with the program started at Thiokol after the *Challenger* disaster, which happened in January that same year.

Thiokol had a plant in Northern Utah, where the solid rocket boosters were tested. As a fellow (senior trainee) in occupational and environmental medicine at the University of Utah, I was invited by the medical director at that plant to spend a day with him learning about the health and safety programs he supervised. He briefed me about the requirements for drug and alcohol testing that had recently been promulgated by Thiokol, affecting every employee at his plant, because starting the program so quickly after the disaster had been all-consuming for him. The memo from the "Republican" floor prompted me to telephone both the Thiokol medical director and a law professor in Utah with whom I'd had conversations about the legal aspects of required drug testing. With the law professor's help, I eventually produced an agenda for a proposed national meeting, which we hoped would be hosted by OSHA, about the difficult medical and legal issues associated with workplace drug and alcohol testing. We spent many hours collaborating on the project and hoped to get the deputy assistant secretary to induce the secretary of labor to endorse the concept and fund the conference.

Evidently, however, the week I took to prepare the agenda was too much time for the deputy assistant secretary to stay focused on one subject, because having lost interest in the whole enterprise, she stopped responding to my phone calls and memos just after I delivered the proposal to her.

That was my first experience with a massive infusion of my time and effort in response to some other person's perception of a political opportunity. Having now, years later, served in government at both the state and federal levels, I know that government bureaucratic inertia is far more massive in Washington, DC. State-elected officials and employees are much closer to the public they serve and much more responsive to constituent needs. Governor John Kasich (R-OH) has written: "We need to take our money, power and influence from Washington and bring it back to the states and communities where we live. That is the federalism the Founding Fathers intended for us."[4] That statement squares well with my own experience.

It began to dawn on me that one should not take every urgent memo seriously. The attention span of many politicians is no longer than a news cycle. Difficult problems, like how to improve health care, cannot be solved one news cycle at a time.

Not long after I started working at OSHA, I was sent (while the weather was still quite warm, unfortunately) to Beaumont, Texas, where OSHA inspectors were carrying out surprise reviews of various large plants. I went to one oil refinery and a chemical plant in order to examine their injury logs. These are the records of work-related injuries American employers are required by OSHA to keep. No one, to my knowledge, had ever cared about these injury logs until after the massive accident at Bhopal, India, which has been called the world's largest industrial disaster.

This event occurred in December 1984. A toxic gas leak exposed 500,000 people with 2,000 immediate and 8,000 subsequent deaths. In the United States, as a reaction to the outpouring of grief over this tragedy, OSHA descended upon Union Carbide's Institute, West Virginia, plant in 1985 and thoroughly scoured everything. They found nothing except alleged violations relating to failure to properly maintain the injury log.

So, apparently in the spirit of trying to be punitive, fines totaling more than $1 million were levied against Union Carbide operations in the United States, which, of course, were challenged in court. Union Carbide's lawyers asserted that these fines, and indeed the entire review of the injury log, were arbitrary and capricious because no other OSHA inspection anywhere had ever focused on the injury log or rendered a fine of any amount for failure to properly keep the log. So OSHA immediately began looking at injury logs all over the nation, and I became a foot soldier in that massive effort.

Typically, I would show up at the security gate of the subject plant and identify myself. In response, the security staff would telephone someone and then return and tell me I would not be admitted to the plant. I would then produce a legal document given me by the OSHA official who had briefed me before I left on the assignment (who had obviously anticipated everything about this curious dance between regulator and regulated) and indicate to the security staff that the document required he admit me to the facility. After a phone consultation, he would open the gate and direct me to the administrative office.

Upon arrival, I would be met by some official looking person who would tell me that while I was admitted to the plant, I would not be allowed access to the medical records and injury log, whereupon I would produce another document with which I had been prearmed, which required I be given the necessary access.

Then I would be told that I could look at the injury log and medical records but could not use their copier, and the dance would go on. Ultimately I would do the review everyone on both sides of the issue knew was bound to happen, which took about a week of my time. In the process, I would become friendly with the people from the plant assigned to be with me (they, like me, were merely carrying out someone else's agenda), and inevitably we would talk and become a bit more relaxed about each other. Before I left the oil refinery, for instance, I took a tour of the entire facility given by my attendant. In fact, I was shown the deep pit into which the refuse from oil refining was being dumped.

Curious, I asked what happened to that chemical mess once it was hundreds of feet down. The answer was that it probably followed a geological layer out under the Gulf of Mexico and would not emerge any closer than five miles offshore. Nothing I saw on the injury log even approached the public-health significance of that finding, but, of course, the pit was not OSHA's concern. No government program I've administered was anywhere near as feckless or uncaring than was the sheer audacity of this private-sector refinery in doing damage to the environment. The government is not always the problem; sometimes it's the solution.

This experience was my first lesson in being politically correct. There was universal (or should I say, bipartisan) anguish about the Bhopal disaster. However, just because Union Carbide failed to protect the people in India did not justify the politically motivated effort to discover something in Union Carbide's US operations for which US government officials could punish the company. The punishment was simply the politically correct thing to do. And even when the fine levied became legally silly, government officials doubled down by looking for similar flaws in the records of other US firms. Meanwhile, real and massive environmental health problems were ignored.

Similarly, what is politically correct in health care "reform" is almost never about correcting or reforming what is really wrong with American health-care delivery. It is politically correct for both Democrats and Republicans to trumpet the market as the solution to health-system woes, yet there is nothing like a market in the distribution of health care.

Halfway through my postgraduate year in Washington, DC, my superiors began making overtures about whether I might consider a permanent position with OSHA. My family was doing well in the Arlington, Virginia, neighborhood where we lived. The schools were excellent, and the kids had made some good friends. But the salary offered was not enough to live comfortably within easy commuting distance to Washington, DC (like Arlington), so we would've had to move anyway. More importantly for me, I really didn't relish the foot-soldier aspect of my work. As often as not, I seemed to be employed in futile exercises supporting enforcement or the agonizingly slow process of writing new standards. In short, I wanted to believe my work would make a difference.

So it was easy to become interested in a job that was posted (I can't remember where) in early 1987: Nevada State health officer.

If I'd had more professional experience, I probably would not have accepted the Nevada job offer. A more experienced public-health physician could see how impossible it would be to affect real change in Nevada's community health. In fact, I believe more experienced public-health physicians actually did pass up this opportunity, which was why the search committee for the state health officer in Nevada in the spring of 1987 was so anxious to make a good impression on me.

The dean of the University of Nevada School of Medicine, Bob Daugherty, took me to dinner the night after my interview with the search committee and asked if I wanted the job, adding that if I did, it was mine for the taking.

I was elated and quite impressed with myself. In hindsight, I should've just accepted the offer from the University of Utah to return to Salt Lake City as junior faculty. But I can't say I regret going to Nevada. I learned more about public health—my professional passion—in just over two years than would have been possible in any other situation. And I made a few good friends, like Dean Daugherty, who kindly mentored me and never abandoned me, even though he came to view me as a most impatient man.

Dr. Daugherty went out of his way to introduce me to some of the more important political figures in the state. But he also tried to warn me about those people.

Politicians, he said repeatedly, could not be trusted. Of course, he was and is correct. Every voter needs to keep that observation foremost. Dishonesty is what makes it possible for politicians to succeed in being repeatedly reelected. We voters have only ourselves to blame for the disingenuous political process. Until we stop electing liars and dissemblers, we will continue to have untrustworthy leaders.

Despite all the signals that should have warned me away, I rashly accepted the job. The day I began serving as Nevada's state health officer in August 1987, I found a postcard report of a case of typhoid fever in a pile of mail on my desk. It seems the mail had been collecting for some time prior to my arrival, apparently without anyone screening it.

Worldwide, there are millions of cases of typhoid fever each year, with about six hundred thousand deaths. It is a bacterial disease characterized by fever, cough, rash, enlargement of the spleen, malaise, headache, and poor appetite. If not treated with an antibiotic, as many as one in five cases will end in death. This typhoid-fever case report represented, for me, a chance to finally engage in a real effort to protect the health of the public, in contrast to what I'd been doing since finishing my training program. I thought I might discover something useful about the function of Nevada's state public-health agency by taking the typhoid fever card down the hall to the communicable-disease program office myself. Though worldwide typhoid fever causes around six hundred thousand deaths every year, less than five hundred cases of typhoid fever happen annually in the United States. If, in fact, a case had occurred, it could be a sentinel event indicating possible contamination of food or water with the feces of a carrier of the bacteria. In public health, this kind of disease transmission is commonly called the fecal-oral route.

And this type of infection transmission is quite common. In fact, it is the quintessential example of the purple world previously mentioned during my microbiological study in medical school.

Public-health agencies are supposed to make the world a little less purple.

It occurred to me that with tens of millions of visitors each year in Nevada, there may be as many meals served in buffet lines and other restaurants as there are served in Nevada homes. These public eating establishments needed protection from bacterial, viral, and other kinds of contamination. Or so I thought.

I walked purposely through a door in the offices of the Nevada State Health Division upon which hung a sign reading "Communicable Disease Control" and encountered a receptionist. I introduced myself and showed her the post card, which had been sent to the "Nevada State Health Division" by a physician in Fallon, a small town about fifty miles east of Carson City, the capital of Nevada. She thanked me and then took the card and filed it in a cabinet next to her desk.

Surprised, I inquired whether anyone would be looking into the case report. She responded that there was no one else besides herself involved with the routine handling of infectious-disease case reports. The two larger counties in Nevada, Washoe and Clark, where, respectively, Reno and Las Vegas are located, have independent local health departments that, to some degree, actually did have paid staff doing traditional communicable-disease investigations. The other fifteen counties in Nevada were entirely dependent upon the Nevada State Health Division for the delivery of public-health services.

She assured me that this report, along with all others received during the month, would be included in the next set of case counts forwarded monthly to the Centers for Disease Control.

I asked her to return the card to me so I could look into the case myself.

Clearly, the state public-health agency didn't typically try to make the smaller counties in Nevada less purple.

Over the next few days, I found time to telephone the office of the reporting physician, where a nurse assured me that the case had been verified with laboratory work. She provided me with the address of the individual whose diagnosis had been reported and told me he had no telephone. So I drove to Fallon and found the mobile home where he'd been living. The door opened after I knocked, and I found myself speaking with the widow of the man who had been reported to have typhoid fever. In fact, much to my chagrin, she had returned from the funeral just a few minutes before my arrival.

She told me her husband recently had a gall bladder operation but never really recovered. None of the history sounded at all like typhoid fever to me. It's true that the chronic carrier state for the bacteria that causes typhoid fever can be associated with biliary tract diseases such as gallstones, but as I discovered, this man probably did not have gall bladder disease.

Puzzled, I found the physician's office and asked to speak with the doctor and review the medical chart. The doctor actually took me to lunch, thanked me for taking an interest in the case report, and told me I was the first public-health official to respond to any of the cases he had documented and reported to the Nevada Division of Health. This was not surprising given what I'd just discovered about the communicable disease program at the state health division.

I told him I'd interviewed the widow and had not heard a history consistent with the diagnosis of typhoid fever. He agreed he was surprised by the diagnosis himself. But he would not have sent in the notification had he not been quite sure of the diagnosis. He then opened the medical chart and allowed me to review it while he told me about the case.

The recently deceased patient had been in the doctor's primary care practice for a couple of years. He'd medically retired due to smoking-related lung problems and had migrated to Fallon, where he could afford to park his mobile home.

Most of the medical encounters documented in the chart had been due to exacerbations of the man's chronic bronchitis. A few weeks before his death, however, this patient had complained of some vague right upper quadrant abdominal discomfort and was referred to the only surgeon in town. The next day, without benefit of any clinical testing for gall bladder disease, he was taken to surgery for removal of the gall bladder, which had not been diseased, according to the surgical pathology report.

Postoperatively, he'd had trouble breathing but had managed to get well enough to go home. However, a few days later he was back in the hospital with more breathing trouble. There, he died.

I asked how any of that fit with a diagnosis of typhoid fever.

In response, the doctor explained to me that he and the surgeon were very concerned that this patient required readmission to the hospital. Neither he nor the surgeon had anticipated the possibility that this patient might have trouble tolerating abdominal surgery, despite the patient's obvious preexisting medical problems. So at the time of readmission, he (the primary care doctor) had run some "tests" on the patient using a new device he'd recently purchased.

The device was alleged to be some kind of electromagnetic "reader" used by attaching leads to the patient's skin, apparently anywhere on the body. After attachment, various "diagnosis cards" were inserted into a slot in the machine, one at a time, each of which would then produce a change in the "current" showing on a gauge located on the face of the machine.

By reading these "current" changes, the doctor was allegedly able to determine what the diagnosis was. And in this case, the patient had to be readmitted to the hospital, according to the reading on this machine, because he had typhoid fever.

No bacterial culture had been attempted because the doctor was entirely sure of the diagnosis based upon the results of this electromagnetic "reading." As far as this physician was concerned, the electromagnetic "reader" ruled out any other diagnosis—even worsening of longstanding chronic bronchitis after general anesthesia for abdominal surgery.

I was stunned by what this doctor told me. I didn't know what to say. I thought perhaps someone would jump from behind a potted plant in the restaurant and shout "You're on *Candid Camera*!"

The whole episode still seems so unreal to me I wonder if I dreamed it up. It made me wonder about what part of the planet had become my home. Was I still in the first world, or had I driven my family clear into the third world? Why weren't the clinical-science methods first articulated by Dr. Hunter being applied in Nevada? The electromagnetic reader machine seemed to hearken back to bloodletting but with a façade of technology. I was the lead public-health official, but I had no staff who could carry out an investigation of a reported typhoid fever case. And I'd begun my first case investigation (actually the first communicable-disease investigation outside Washoe and Clark Counties in decades) by disturbing a widow fresh home from the mortuary. And then I'd met an enthusiastic physician who told me all about his wondrous new diagnostic machine, which was patently devoid of any science.

He had referred a patient to have surgery based only upon a report of vague abdominal symptoms. And a surgeon had operated on that poor man without confirming a diagnosis. He and the surgeon had failed to consider the possible complications of taking a patient with chronic lung problems to the operating room and were, in fact, surprised when the patient did not do well. Fallon is less than five hundred miles from Salt

Lake City, where I received my medical degree and completed residencies in family medicine and public health. But during my first business lunch as state health officer of Nevada, I felt far removed from the clinical science I'd learned in Utah. Fallon is located on US Highway 50, which has often been dubbed "The Loneliest Highway in America." I sure felt professionally lonely alongside that highway that particular day. It began to dawn on me that the world could be purple for reasons other than microbiological exposure.

In fact, as is illustrated by this case, in the United States, our population is at far greater risk from injury by the health-care delivery system than it is from fecal-oral contamination. Preventable injury to hospitalized patients is a leading cause of death in the United States, as has been studied multiple times by the Institute of Medicine, a nonpartisan, nonprofit organization that examines health-policy problems in the United States. I commonly tell friends and family to never leave their loved ones alone in the hospital because that is where they are most vulnerable. I've heard it said that if the safety record of American hospitals were to be superimposed upon the airline industry, a fully loaded 747 would crash every other week. The preeminent purple world for the average American is when he or she steps into the American health-care system as a patient.

To be fair, this problem is not unique to Nevada. During my training in Salt Lake City, I'd seen a number of egregious surgical interventions. One I still regret was the case of a woman in her early thirties who visited with a general surgeon because of pelvic pain. And, like in Fallon, without benefit of any diagnostic workup, the surgeon admitted her to a hospital (where I was a third-year medical student on a required general-surgery rotation) in preparation for surgery, specifically hysterectomy and bilateral salpingo-oopherectomy (she was to have her uterus and both ovaries removed).

I was assigned to do her admitting history and physical examination. Having just completed a gynecology rotation at the same hospital, I knew the proposed surgery was premature at best, and that in any case, the removal of both ovaries was not indicated. She was too young to be forced into surgical menopause. The patient herself had no notion that she was being poorly advised. (In fact, patients make poor "buyers" in a health-care "market" because they almost never know what they need to purchase nor what constitutes a high-quality "product" in health care. They believe what their doctor tells them, even if, as in this case, the doctor would rather make a "sale" than care for the patient.) I left her bedside and went to the medical library, where I copied a couple of articles documenting that the removal of the ovaries was not appropriate and showed them to the attending surgeon.

He took an aggressive stance with me, insisting that many other articles could be cited in support of the proposed surgery (he never produced any). Further, he found my interference with this case to be highly inappropriate for a mere medical student. I asked to be allowed to withdraw, but he indicated that he would arrange for me to receive a failing grade for the required surgical course if I did not participate fully and with no further attempts to influence his chosen clinical interventions.

Dutifully, the next day I was in the operating room and watched while he butchered the case. There was no other way to describe what happened. I'd seen many hysterectomies while studying gynecology. The procedure, done correctly, is remarkably quick, with minimal blood loss. This general surgeon hadn't done a hysterectomy in who knows how long, if ever. He had almost no idea about the anatomy, and he was being assisted by the chief surgical resident, who was very capable but had never done a hysterectomy either. Dr. Hunter would have been appalled by the whole episode.

Still, without the chief resident's great surgical instincts and hands, the patient would have died on the operating-room table. She lost five units of blood before the organ was removed. It was awful. The next morning, I was performing my rounds when I happened to be at her bedside at the same time she was visited by the attending surgeon. He laid claim to having saved her life during the surgery the day before. That too was a surreal and lonely (and purple) moment. (These types of purple moments are what can be called "quality waste" in American health care.

These happen routinely, unfortunately, and are in three general categories: (a) inappropriate care, such as in this case, when there is no real clinical indication for an intervention; (b) preventable patient injury, also such as in this case; and (c) failing to do what is generally known to be indicated by published and accepted clinical science. Quality waste costs the American health-care system more than $700 billion dollars annually.)

But that case at the hospital in Salt Lake City was an exception. In contrast, my time in Nevada was studded with surreal moments. I'm not the first person to have remarked about the difference between Utah and Nevada when it comes to health. In his book entitled *Who Shall Live,* Victor R. Fuchs (now a professor at Stanford University) observed:

> In the western United States, there are two contiguous states that enjoy about the same levels of income and medical care and are alike in many other respects, but their levels of health differ enormously. The inhabitants of Utah are among the healthiest individuals in the United States, while the residents of Nevada are at the opposite end of the spectrum. Comparing death rates of white residents in the two states, for example, we find that infant mortality is about 40 percent higher in Nevada. . . . The excess mortality . . . differential for adult men and women is in the range of 40 to 50 percent. . . . The two states are very much alike with respect to income, schooling, degree of urbanization, climate, and many other variables that are frequently thought to be the cause of variations in mortality. . . . What, then, explains these huge differences in death rates? The answer almost surely lies in the different lifestyles of the residents of the two states. Utah is inhabited primarily by Mormons, whose influence is strong throughout the state. Devout Mormons do not use tobacco or alcohol and in general lead stable, quiet lives. Nevada, on the other hand, is a state with high rates of cigarette and alcohol consumption and very high indexes of marital and geographical instability. The contrast with Utah in these respects is extraordinary. . . . The populations of these two states are, to a considerable extent, self-selected extremes

from the continuum of lifestyles found in the United States. Nevadans . . . are predominantly recent immigrants from other areas,
many of whom were attracted by the state's permissive mores. The
inhabitants of Utah, on the other hand, are evidently willing to
remain in a more restricted society. Persons born in Utah who do
not find these restrictions acceptable tend to move out of the state.[5]

Before I agree with Professor Fuchs's characterization of the health
and habits of Nevadans, allow me to disagree with his notion that Mormonism makes Utah a more "restricted" society that is a "self-selected
extreme" along the continuum of American lifestyle. I'm not a native of
Utah. I was born in Tucson and raised in Phoenix, but I am a seventh-gen-
eration Mormon with family ties to Utah. I lived in Utah prior to becoming the Nevada state health officer while I earned my college degree
(BA-English, BYU, 1978) and undertook my professional training (MD
and MSPH-University of Utah, 1982 and 1986). In addition to Utah and
Nevada, I have lived in Arizona, Virginia, and Colorado. There are more
Mormons in Nevada than there are in Virginia and Colorado combined,
and Mormons compose a higher percentage of the population in Nevada
than in Arizona. In fact, Las Vegas was originally a Mormon settlement
and still has a substantial population of Latter-day Saints. (The name of
this religion is actually The Church of Jesus Christ of Latter-day Saints. It
is commonly called the Mormon Church because of the church's acceptance of the Book of Mormon as scripture.)

There are now enough Mormons in both Reno and Las Vegas for the
leadership of the LDS Church to locate a temple in each city. A temple is
a building for special worship reserved for devout members of the faith,
principally adults, and is different from the far more common chapels or
regular church buildings built for Sunday worship services and community events. There are about 150 temples throughout the world, but about
one hundred times that many chapels. Mormons are not so uncommon
in Nevada as Professor Fuchs may have thought. Members of the faith are
not overwhelmingly self-selecting out of Nevada and into Utah.

Nor are Mormons an "extreme" along the continuum of American lifestyles. We (Mormons) are commonly the objects of caricature on the stage and screen, in the news, and often in academic pronouncements (such as this one from Professor Fuchs). It is true that, unlike many, we eschew the consumption of recreational drugs, alcohol, tobacco, and coffee. And we maintain that old-fashioned family values are best and therefore strive to live chaste lives characterized by sexual abstinence before marriage and fidelity to spouse thereafter. We also tithe ourselves, fast once each month, generously donate time and money to the poor, and accept personal responsibility for participating in the lay ministry that serves our congregations. But these devotions, rather than being on the extreme of American culture, are the full fruition of an American passion for biblical living that has dominated the American way of life since the Pilgrims, certainly up to the 1970s, when Professor Fuchs was first writing his book. To the extent that individual Mormons succeed in adhering to these virtues, they are blessed with better health, and their communities are favored with reduced poverty and loneliness. How is that anything other than the flowering of the goodness of the American spirit? How is it that Professor Fuchs refers to this as a restrictive lifestyle instead of recognizing the freedom from illness and want of social support that Mormonism encourages wherever it is practiced?

Perhaps I've said enough about Professor Fuchs's backhanded compliment regarding the healthiness of Mormon life. But the awkwardness of his statement and the lingering anti-Mormon bias it reflects has touched me in personal and professional ways throughout my career. But for the fact that I'm a Mormon, I probably would have had at least two other opportunities to lead state or local health agencies. I was a finalist for such a position in Colorado a few years after I left Nevada. As such, I was invited to meet then governor Roy Romer (D-CO), who took one look at my CV, saw the reference to my undergraduate university (BYU), and asked, "Are you a Mormon?"

When Governor Romer heard my response to his inappropriate question about my faith, he made a comment about Mormonism being a poor fit for public health, but would I consider serving on the Gaming Control Board? Casino gambling had just been legalized by voter referendum in Colorado, over Governor Romer's objections, and the governor was trying to fill seats on the newly created board with people unfriendly to gaming. Mormons are taught to not gamble. In fact, Utah is perhaps the only state that allows no form of legalized gambling. People who favor gaming know that Mormons are not players, though it is often said in Nevada that casino owners love to employ Mormons because they can be trusted with the large volumes of cash that flow through those establishments.

It's probably true that my personal opposition to gaming would have isolated me from those with the most political influence in Nevada had we ever been introduced. During the three years I lived in Nevada, I never gambled, not even a nickel, though I spent many hours inside gambling establishments (mostly at various conferences). Unlike Professor Fuchs's characterization (and the assumptions of many who are by nature or choice more "permissive"), however, I was not entering Nevada full of religious zeal from the extreme of the continuum of American lifestyle with intent to call gamblers and other sinners to repentance.

I came with an understanding that public health must operate within the society it tries to serve, and I intended to accept what was legal, not change it. I was told that the state of Nevada had made a policy decision to hire a state health officer (for the first time in several years) because of a perception that poor health among the citizenry was excessive and could be improved. And should be improved, because better community health is a societal asset. In his book, Professor Fuchs correctly states both that poor health is generally not a random event and that Nevadans as a group had the poorest health among Americans. What he did not perceive from a distance was how irrelevant public-health policy could be in Nevada. I was never introduced to the political power players in Nevada's gaming industry because they really could not have cared less about public health. It was simply irrelevant to their business interests, as events in my tenure as state health officer proved, at least to me. In the high-stakes poker game of public policy about the health of Nevadans, I was not dealt a hand because I wasn't even in the smoke-filled back room where the cards were being shuffled.

Some who tend to be secular try to exclude people of faith, like myself, from health policy because they find an inevitable conflict between the values of religion and the facts of science. Personally, I see no such conflict. Religion and science are two synergistic ways to understand the human condition. Others who are business-oriented do their best to exclude anyone from public policy discussions who might have the notion that business interests (meaning optimizing profit) should not always be the principle object of public policy. The values of religion and the facts of science are both in conflict with that viewpoint. I'm not opposed to making money, but business interests do not take precedence over human life and health.

Business leaders in the private, for-profit health-care sector have a fiduciary duty to their stockholders to make as much money as possible. They don't have an obligation to patients to provide the best health care possible. Because of the nature of health care, best-quality care is not only optimal for the patient, it's less expensive and therefore less profitable. For-profit health-care businesses exploit episodes of pathology for profit. They are not required to do what is best for patients. This is essentially the cause of the purple world in American health care.

Chapter Three

Prostitution and Health Insurance— The Similarities

N EVADA IS A caricature of the American free-enterprise concept. Everywhere else in the United States, citizens have tended to come to a kind of consensus about what is good and right and just, and we bless those activities with a legal status. Once a product or service is considered legal, free enterprise kicks in and the door is open for those who wish to make money producing these goods and services to do so. But, in Nevada, the initial judgment made about goods and services is not whether they should be legal but whether they might be profitable. If profitable, then they are inevitably made legal.

I'm an endorser of free enterprise as the most efficient means to distribute goods and services. However, I came to thoroughly dislike the Nevada distortion of market economics, because it's deployed at a societal cost.

During my tenure in Nevada, gaming was the principle industry in the state and was not generally found elsewhere in the United States. To be a successful politician in Nevada required catering to the gaming interests. This created confusing politics in Nevada. With both parties vying for favor from gaming leaders, there was often no perceptible policy difference between candidates. Or, in modern American political parlance, you couldn't tell the difference between the red and blue candidates—which gives a different meaning to the purple-world metaphor.

Some candidates are selected not so much for ability as for fidelity to gambling. That must have been the case with Senator Chick Hecht (R-NV), who was serving his first and only term in the US Senate (along with then fellow first-termer but eventually much longer tenured and now-retired Harry Reid, D-NV) when I learned I would be moving to their home state.

Senator Hecht has now passed away, and some would say I should hesitate to demean the dead. But the fact is that in the 1980s, he was termed the worst-serving US senator by the *New York Times*. My personal exposure to him consisted of going to his office in Washington, DC, before I moved to Nevada to introduce myself. I'd made an appointment and so was met by his staff and placed in a small room, much like three others who had come for appointments at the same time. After a few minutes, the senator came into the room smiling mechanically and already moving his hand up and down in handshake fashion and mumbling "So nice to see you" over and over.

And then he left, presumably to repeat that scene in the next room. His staff person apologized for the inadequate meeting and asked me for some information about the reason for my visit. Just as I was beginning to respond, the senator returned to the room and repeated exactly what he had done not five minutes before. This time the staff member was so obviously embarrassed that there was nothing more to say, and he simply showed me the door.

I met a number of people in public office in Nevada, both elected and appointed, with not much more than that same level of competence. True, incompetence and worse is commonly associated with public officials all across the nation. But only the US senator from Nevada was designated the worst by the *New York Times*. As perverse as this may sound, however, Senator Hecht's incompetence was actually better for the American public than is the would-be competence of any member of Congress whose only purpose is to manipulate the electoral process long enough to become personally wealthy and/or achieve some other self-aggrandizement.

"Competent" politicians, unlike Senator Hecht, get reelected and continue to ignore the needs of the American people while feathering their own nests through assisting corporate interests.

In the long run, which first-term senator (in 1987) from Nevada did the most harm to the American people: Senator Hecht, who was judged the worst senator of his era by the *New York Times* and failed to be reelected, or Senator Harry Reid, who rose to US Senate majority leader and helped President Obama ram through the Patient Protection and Affordable Care Act? (Obamacare, in my opinion, makes everything that is bad about American health care worse.) I acknowledge that it's unfair to judge Senator Reid, who is a practicing Mormon, solely on his support of Obamacare. So, by way of providing balance, let me note that Mitt Romney, also a practicing Mormon, was equally guilty of legislating harm when he signed Romneycare into law in Massachusetts in 2006. I believe I've cast ballots for both men.

Sometimes, when a particularly repugnant but profitable enterprise is made legal, or kept indefinitely not illegal, by the unique Nevada political paradigm, an effort is needed to fashion a more palatable public image. These efforts are inevitably successful because Nevadans as a group are good at looking the other way. High rates of death and disease, as documented by Professor Fuchs, are not really enough to generate much interest in obstructing profit-making enterprises.

For example, Nevada is infamously the only American state where prostitution is legal. Or, more accurately stated, where prostitution is not illegal. But the "not-illegal" status applies only to brothels located in counties other than Washoe (where Reno is located) and Clark (where Las Vegas is located). Individual prostitutes cannot do business on their own. The brothel owner provides the only venue allowed. Local government agencies provide these brothel owners with business licenses. There has not been a state effort to regulate this industry. Local law enforcement in small-town Nevada (which can be very small) is necessarily quite subject to the influence of the local "business" owners. It doesn't take much imagination to perceive that a brothel can be a place of exploitation.

As I understood the business of prostitution in Nevada, the women were not employees of, but independent contractors with, the brothel owners. They could be terminated at any time and tossed out of the "house." As independent contractors, they were required to pay for the supplies and facilities they used. The prostitutes received some portion of the fee charged by the brothel for the "service" of customers, and out of that portion, these women would pay rent for the room, fees for laundry, and charges for supplies of food and presumably toilet paper. Whatever was left was theirs, after they made the necessary arrangements for federal tax withholding.

At least the state of Nevada had no income tax subtracting even more from their bottom line (sorry for the pun). A woman who, for whatever reason, failed to satisfy the brothel owner might find herself on the street of a very small place with not a friend between her and the horizon. Or worse. Off-the-record accounts told me by emergency-room personnel indicated that not so rarely there would be violently abused women dropped off for treatment with costs covered in cash. I can't verify any of this.

I've never visited a brothel. I was invited to participate in a national TV discussion about Nevada brothel prostitution once, which was to be staged at a brothel. I think the show was to be hosted by Geraldo Rivera. I turned the opportunity down. I don't think there's anything to gain by assuming there's something about Nevada brothels worth seriously discussing.

Brothel industry representatives will present a different image of their enterprise, of course. They like to style themselves as entrepreneurs serving the basic needs of society. Monogamy, they say, has its societal value. But it's not practical because the human male is promiscuous by nature. And so, the brothel proponents argue, there's a legitimate need for a sexual outlet, but one without the messy complications of passionate peccadilloes among one's neighbors. The brothel owners claim to recruit women who could be your neighbors (waitresses, housewives, college students) to provide a personal service for pay, a source of income much needed by these allegedly otherwise virtuous girls. And further, they claim that the john's significant others (wives and girlfriends) are delighted to have a night off without fear of their man becoming entangled with the girl next door.

It seems most Nevadans are willing to go along with this burnished image, or at least not care if there may be a seamier side. Allegations of kidnapping, enslavement, IV drug abuse, and deployment of underage girls have been made but not seriously investigated.

But then, in the 1980s, something really fearful crept into that picture: AIDS.

Acquired immune deficiency syndrome was the highest profile disease throughout the nation by the time I accepted an appointment to serve as the Nevada state health officer in 1987. The Reagan administration tried to ignore the disease. In fact, President Reagan refused to speak about HIV or AIDS in public until Surgeon General C. Everett Coop masterfully brought the issue front and center for public discussion. His publication of an AIDS pamphlet written for the general public caught the White House by surprise and fashioned out of him a public-health icon. By then it was well established that unprotected sexual intercourse and intravenous drug use were the principle pathways to HIV infection. Nonetheless, there was a floating anxiety everywhere in the United States that other pathways were possible (for instance, some people in Florida were persuaded the disease could be spread by mosquitoes).

People with HIV (the virus that causes AIDS) infection commonly kept their health condition secret for fear of mistreatment, or, more accurately said, no treatment, because it was not uncommon for doctors and nurses to refuse to lay a hand on HIV-infected patients. Naturally, in the face of such fear, the Nevada brothel industry realized it had a potential public-relations problem. Even one report of HIV in a prostitute would ruin business. So, a few months before I arrived in Carson City to assume my new duties, all of the brothels in Nevada made a public commitment to test every woman working in a brothel every month for HIV, or at least said they would do so.

I remember seeing the results of the first month's tests published in the *Washington Post* while I still lived in Arlington, Virginia, prior to moving my family west. Not surprisingly, the brothels failed to find a single HIV-positive woman working as a prostitute. After all, didn't they only employ (or technically, contract with) the sweet girls next door? Month after month, ever since then (for more than a quarter of a century) the brothel industry issued HIV test results without ever finding a woman who was HIV positive. How blissful it must be to do public relations in a state with citizens so willingly credulous.

But then, the American public is just as willingly credulous when it comes to our health-care system. We are told, and Americans by and large accept, that we have the world's best health care. Yet American health care costs vastly more than health care delivered anywhere else in the world. Whether measured on a per-capita basis or as a percentage of the gross domestic product, the cost of American health care is about twice that of the average first-world country. And yet we're arguably less well-served by our health-care system and therefore less healthy. Numerous credible sources indicate that this gap in annual health-care spending between the United States and other developed nations is due to about $1 trillion in wasteful spending. That means business as usual in American health care is throwing away $1 trillion each year. What is the opportunity cost of these losses?

What could we be doing with that $1 trillion each year? Most of the money in American health care is tax money. Americans pay more taxes for health care, by far, than do the citizens of any other country. Therefore, many hundreds of billions of tax dollars supposedly destined for public health-care services are wasted. This waste is mostly due to poor-quality care, as noted previously. But there is also a significant loss due to the inefficiency of our unique American health-care financing business model for providing health insurance. As much as $400 billion per year is wasted on the useless overhead of health insurers.

How many children could be educated? How many roads built or repaired? How many tax rebates granted? And what would American taxpayers do with hundreds of billions of dollars annually? How much GDP growth have we lost through wasteful health-system spending?

And yet, when American politicians of either party talk about American health care, they always say we have the world's best health-care system. The reality is that we pay through the nose for a wasteful system that is least able (among first-world countries) to prevent deaths that should be amenable to health-care interventions. Obviously, American politicians are telling the American people what they want to hear, never mind the abysmal performance of American health care. It's like wanting to believe there has never been a prostitute in Nevada in three decades who was infected with HIV.

Not long after the brothels began the practice of HIV testing, and just about the time I arrived in Nevada, a blue-ribbon committee was established to review Nevada state policy concerning HIV and AIDS. If I remember correctly, it was named the AIDS Task Force. There were several well-informed, highly concerned citizens on this committee, and their work was highly credible (something remarkable for blue-ribbon committees anywhere, and any kind of policy committee ever in Nevada). The task force was formed and had already met once before I arrived in Carson City. It was co-chaired by one member each from the Nevada State Senate and State Assembly, and staffed by Larry Matheis, the administrator of the Nevada Division of Health. Matheis was also my immediate superior.

Larry's predecessor had been dismissed with the general acknowledgment that the state health division was underperforming, and Larry was given the job of cleaning it up and making public health relevant. He frankly acknowledged to me that he had no training or experience in public health. So he'd scraped together from various budgets the requisite ongoing funding to pay a state health officer salary (not much even for a public-health physician and perhaps the more important reason why more experienced candidates before me had refused the job). Larry worked to get the governor and legislature to include the position in the biennial budget passed in 1987. By way of telling me about this accomplishment, he was informing me that his forte was political leadership, which he considered his domain at the health division. He was looking for a public-health physician who would join him as a partner in forming the public-health science half of the health-agency leadership team.

He couldn't promise to get the political system in Nevada to consistently support public-health science, but he did promise me he'd never allow me to be taken by surprise. For my part, he asked me to never let him wade into an issue uninformed about public-health science.

In the spirit of this "no surprises" partnership, Larry asked me to remain on the sidelines as his adviser during the AIDS Task Force. This was a legislative task force, meaning it was specifically designed to launch bill drafts into the 1989 legislative session. Given how anxiety-provoking the issues related to HIV and AIDS already were, these bill drafts would have a decent chance at passage. Nevada was late among the states in formulating a response to the AIDS epidemic (no surprise there), meaning there was a sense of urgency that something must be done.

So the task force was likely a target for all kinds of potential seekers of legislative favor who would love to hang their ornaments on this holiday tree. Larry intended to remain firmly in control of who got close enough to this enterprise so that he could prevent the hanging of cheap tinsel. He was right to sense that I was a political novice. And he kept his word: he never allowed me to be surprised by what happened at the task-force meetings, or anywhere else, for that matter.

Larry also knew that the brothel industry was desperate to hang their cheap tinsel on that AIDS Task Force tree. He was savvy enough to realize that he could not entirely prevent their efforts to have their image burnished by the good work of the AIDS Task Force. They wanted an opportunity to share in the public spotlight shining on the task force work by testifying at one of the several scheduled hearings. Larry didn't want the brothel industry to muck up any proposed legislation by getting language of their own into a bill draft. And the brothel industry did not want any language in legislation that might actually require them to submit to real public-health surveillance.

So he struck a compromise with the brothel association. They were allowed to testify at the task-force hearing if they would limit themselves to asking only for rules about the testing of prostitutes to be considered and passed by the state board of health and not ask the task force to sponsor prostitution-related legislation.

The rules the brothel owners proposed were, of course, self-serving. They asked the Nevada Board of Health to "regulate" by "requiring" what they were already doing: 1) the monthly testing of all brothel prostitutes for HIV, syphilis, and gonorrhea and 2) requiring the use of condoms in the brothels.

But the rules specified that the brothels themselves were in charge of enforcement. The fox was officially in charge of henhouse hygiene (sorry, another bad pun), but now with the imprimatur of the Nevada Board of Health. The regulations provided for no oversight and no penalties. The only thing that changed in the "business" of running a brothel was that the independent contractors (the prostitutes) now had monthly lab costs to pay for. Larry was politically correct enough to hold his nose and agree to this bargain in order to get the brothels out of the real public-health work needing attention from the AIDS Task Force. And I was grateful he protected me from direct involvement with the rule-making exercise related to the sham regulation of brothels.

And it is a sham. Prostitution is legal in many countries around the world, and this is decidedly not how public-health surveillance of prostitutes is organized and conducted. In an effort to shed the light of clinical science on public-health surveillance of prostitution, and in response to a private request for information from the state senator who co-chaired the AIDS Task Force (Ray Rawson, R-LV, who became a personal friend and who is also a Mormon), I used the then new technology offered by the National Library of Medicine (now evolved into an easily used online tool called PubMed) to search the world's published, peer-reviewed medical literature for data about how to conduct medical screenings in the sex industry.

As far as I know, I introduced the concept of basing public-health policy on published evidence to the state of Nevada. I was aware of only one other person in the entire state in 1987 with master's-degree-level training in public health. No one even seemed able to pronounce the word *epidemiology,* and there had never been a state epidemiologist, ever. But I repeat myself about the insignificance of public health in Nevada.

The literature search concerning medical surveillance for prostitutes indicated that nothing about the Nevada way of doing things would reduce sexually transmitted disease among the women and their customers. To be effective, according to the published experience of public-health authorities worldwide, there should be no barriers, financial or otherwise, between the women and the public-health services they needed. All of the fifteen or so known sexually transmitted diseases should be included in the screening protocol, not just a selected few. (The most common STD in Nevada in 1987 was chlamydia, which inexplicably was not included in the "regulations" governing STD surveillance in Nevada brothels.)

The purpose of the screening should have been to assure that the women received all the health-care services they needed. Those with disease should be offered treatment without regard to ability to pay.

And if the apparent approval of public health was to be placed on the program, there should have been a direct connection between public-health services and the women themselves, allowing the public-health departments to verify that every woman was being appropriately screened and treated. This included verifying that the laboratory and clinical services used were competent. None of these essential features was true of the sham prostitution regulations in Nevada.

Data that I found in the records of the Nevada Health Division from before the discovery of HIV and AIDS in the United States documented that brothel prostitutes had been tested for syphilis and gonorrhea for many years, roughly on a monthly basis. The incidence of gonorrhea infection had been six hundred cases per one thousand women per year, likely for decades. I doubt there has ever been a group of women with a higher annual incidence of gonorrhea. Brothels are truly part of the purple world.

Why should anyone assume that just because the brothel owners promised universal condom use there would suddenly be an end to the transmission of STDs in brothels? Apparently, gullible men came to Nevada brothels with exactly that expectation. I received a number of anonymous calls complaining that I was doing a poor job as state health officer because the caller had acquired an STD in a brothel (usually chlamydia). My response was always the same: sexual promiscuity is risky behavior, and don't let anyone's advertising tell you otherwise.

Here, there is another striking parallel between Nevada brothel business and the business of health care in the United States. Just as the regulation of brothel health is a sham in Nevada, so was the regulation of the business practices of American health insurers under Obamacare. The basic deal of Obamacare, or so the American public was led to believe, was that individuals were required to buy health insurance or pay a penalty, and in exchange for that odious requirement (health insurance is a hated commodity), insurers were required to issue a policy to all persons who made an application. Now, despite literally thousands of pages of regulations built upon the two thousand pages of the original act of Congress, American consumers are still being jerked around by health-insurance companies. What good does it do an American patient who finally "gets" to buy health insurance if the insurer refuses to contract for services with the only providers nearby who can take care of that patient? Or what about the patient who buys health insurance but then can't afford the copayments and coinsurance? The pretense of coverage through American health insurance is as good as the pretense of health protection in a Nevada brothel—both worlds are deep purple. The proposals so far under Trumpcare, while doing away with the mandate to buy health insurance, make obtaining health care even when insured even more costly for patients.

There came another colorful episode in my experience with brothel prostitution—what I call the "Sally Pink" episode, which particularly illustrates the problems inherent in public-health surveillance as pretense. The Nevada State Laboratory called me to report a case of gonorrhea. The specimen had been submitted by a particular Nevada brothel, and the name on the specimen was "Sally Pink." All STDs are on the list of infectious diseases that must be reported to a health department, both in Nevada and elsewhere in the United States. A report of a sexually transmitted disease is generally followed by a case contact investigation.

The person who has the disease (the case) is treated and interviewed with particular attention to acquiring information about sexual contacts. Those people are then examined, interviewed, and treated. And the people with whom they have had sexual contact are likewise found, etc. Therefore, I asked a public-health nurse located near that particular brothel to find "Sally Pink" and begin case contacting.

The brothel was uncooperative. They denied they knew anyone named Sally Pink. And even if they had known her, they made it clear they'd never allow any case contacting among their clientele. Knowing that many of the men who frequented brothels believed that such behavior carried no STD risk, I felt an imperative to at least give them a chance to find out otherwise, particularly those men who may have had exposure to Sally Pink.

I was especially concerned about the health of the secondary sexual contacts of these men, by which I mean their wives and significant others. So I fashioned a press release identifying the subject brothel by name (I can't remember now which brothel it was, and it really doesn't matter) and indicating a time frame based upon the date of the specimen and the known natural history of gonococcal infection, during which sexual activity at that brothel may have been associated with exposure to the infection. Individuals with possible exposure were advised to seek medical care, and a health division phone number was offered where anonymous information could be obtained.

Larry Matheis gave his approval, and we sent the statement to the usual news outlets. To my surprise, I was inundated with calls for interviews. That evening, this item led the news on the TV station I watched in Reno. My mother, who happened to be visiting that week, saw the story and heard a reporter interview me on camera about STDs. She exclaimed, "I did not raise my son to be speaking about brothels in public!"

The next morning, the Reno newspaper had the story on the front page (above the fold, if I remember correctly), which I read before going to the monthly meeting of the Nevada State Board of Health.

Prior to the meeting, the chairman of the board of health, a local dentist, took me aside and thoroughly chastised me for issuing the press release. He was angry that anyone would make a "big deal" about gonorrhea. "The clap," he said. "You're making a big deal about the clap. Doesn't everyone get the clap sometime in their life? Isn't it just part of growing up?"

He went on to remind me that he had been Governor Bryan's room-mate in college, that he had the governor's personal phone number, and that he would dial that number later in the day to ask the governor to fire me. Another surreal Nevada moment. The chairman of the state board of health considered gonorrhea to be a trivial occurrence and wanted me fired because I disagreed.

He needn't have worried about whether brothel business would be permanently harmed by the fear of gonococci. Subsequent similar news releases drew less and less attention, eventually not making the news at all. It seemed no one cared or noted that if it were possible to acquire any one of the fifteen sexually transmitted diseases at a Nevada brothel, surely HIV could be transmitted there as well, no matter what official test results otherwise indicated. As I said, Nevadans are particularly good at looking the other way when it comes to their peculiar institutions. But in this case, their tolerance was, and continues to be, life-threatening. Likewise, the American health-insurance industry always lands on its feet. They make money no matter who is in office. The rules of American health policy are always in their favor, even though their business prac-tices are life-threatening.

After the Sally Pink case, the state laboratory rarely received any spec-imens for testing from any brothel. After all, the regulations allowed the brothels a completely free hand in choosing where the required testing would be conducted, and they certainly didn't want to have the odd pos-itive specimen reported to the state health division, thereby disrupting business again. But prior thereto, it was not uncommon for many of the brothels to send blood samples to the state laboratory for HIV testing. It was my impression then that the samples were somehow prescreened by the brothels, allowing them a chance to identify and eliminate any HIV-positive specimens.

This practice would assure that HIV-positive blood was never sub-mitted to the state laboratory, or any laboratory, allowing the persistence of the myth of AIDS-free prostitution in Nevada. Likewise, oversight of health insurers under Obamacare was lax or nonexistent. They were free to go on pretending they were offering a worthwhile product at a reasonable price, even though annual price increases were steep.

I decided to test the assertion that the women who worked in Nevada's brothels were free of exposure to infectious disease that, like HIV, would be transmitted by percutaneous or permucosal penetrance of infective blood and body fluids (another part of the purple world). In other words, it was my theory that the women in the Nevada brothels, like prostitutes on the streets of any major American city, were commonly infected with HIV or other blood/body-fluid-borne communicable diseases (like hepatitis B) both because of unprotected, promiscuous sexual activity and because they were IV drug abusers.

So I had the state laboratory test the brothel blood samples for the presence of hepatitis B surface antigen (HBsAg), which is an indicator of potential infectivity for this virus. I didn't ask for official permission to conduct this study, and I directed the laboratory technician involved to keep the results confidential, releasing them only to me.

If I remember correctly, the percentage of brothel prostitute blood specimens that came out positive for HBsAg was about 15 percent, much higher than the rate of chronic hepatitis B infection common in North America (0.5 percent) and very similar to rates documented among prostitutes worldwide. It is, I believe, highly unlikely that a population of sexually promiscuous women with that high of a rate of hepatitis-B surface-antigen positivity would never—in twenty-five years—have a case of HIV infection.

I was naive to think the hepatitis-B results would not be leaked. A woman serving in the Nevada assembly from the Reno area who was also an outspoken critic of Nevada brothels (one of very few) somehow found out about the data. During an assembly Ways and Means Committee hearing in 1989, she asked me whether I had information about blood-borne infectious diseases other than HIV among brothel prostitutes.

I replied as briefly as I could to her questions about the data. I don't think she realized the political peril her question imposed on me. The speaker of the assembly was also a member of that committee. He represented one of the few rural districts in Nevada and was an important legislative ally of the brothels. After the hearing, he immediately buttonholed me and told me that if I ever again conducted research like that, he would personally arrange for me to lose my job.

Another surreal Nevada moment: the speaker of the Nevada assembly cared a great deal about the business interests of brothels and not at all about the health consequences of hepatitis B, a leading cause of chronic liver disease and liver cancer. But that is obviously true of American politicians when it comes to health care. They protect business interests at the expense of patients.

Threats like that were a relatively common occurrence for me during my tenure as state health officer in Nevada. But it's likely that state public-health officials across the country field objections to their policies and priorities often. During a meeting of the Association of State and Territorial Health Officials (ASTHO) I attended as the Nevada state health officer, someone said that the average duration in office for a lead state health official in the United States at that time was about two years.

One cannot be serving the public interest in public health without making some people angry. I developed a sense of purpose as I served, which helped my fortitude under this kind of barrage. I felt I could either try to *do* my job or try to *keep* my job, but I likely would not be able to do both.

Fortunately for me, and unfortunately for those who wished to threaten me, it wasn't easy to get me fired. I'd been hired as a civil servant, not as a political appointee. After I passed my six-month review, neither the governor nor the director of the Nevada Department of Human Resources (the appointing authority for my position) could simply fire me. My job was protected by civil-service statutes and regulations. It was nearly the case that, short of embezzling funds or committing some other intentional malfeasance, they were stuck with me. So I endured longer than either the chairman of the state board of health or the speaker of the Nevada assembly preferred.

I suppose this is like the American people being stuck with Congress term after term, though every poll indicates that US citizens hold

Congress in low esteem. The difference is that there's no civil-service law that keeps the membership of Congress stable. We the people of the United States, who claim to loathe Congress, keep reelecting our own congressman. We are so inclined (through apathy?) to vote on a partisan basis, if we vote at all, that the vast majority of congressional districts are distinctly and repeatedly red or blue. Very few seats in Congress are actually contested in purple districts (the good kind of purple).

Back in Nevada, the brothel association was not content to dislike my service and yet not do anything about it. They took their threats to get rid of me to what, initially, felt like a more serious level. Larry Matheis had been invited to speak at a meeting of the brothel association. For some reason I can't now remember, he was unavailable on the date of the meeting and asked me to stand in for him. This was to be a routine discussion of the board of health regulations requested by the brothels. The meeting took place at Cabin in the Sky, a restaurant located not far from Virginia City, Nevada, and owned by Joe Conforte, owner of the Mustang Ranch. Mr. Conforte himself was not in attendance, though he had been released from federal prison a few years earlier after serving less than two years of a twenty-year sentence.

Unfortunately, the timing of the meeting with the state brothel association was not ideal, at least from my perspective, since it occurred not long after the "Sally Pink" press release. I'd planned a short presentation, but immediately after I began speaking, I was interrupted with questions from the audience. I don't remember finishing more than a sentence or two without interruption for the remainder of my presentation. Many of the interruptions were long tirades from brothel owners who were angry with me because of the approach I'd taken to STD control as exemplified by the "Sally Pink" episode.

I suppose I can see their reasoning. They had, after all, been operating brothels for years with very high rates of gonorrhea, which were known to the Nevada Division of Health, and no one had ever issued a press release before. Because I had the temerity (they would say stupidity) to stick with the principles and facts of public-health science, every answer I gave just made the crowd angrier.

After a couple of hours (by then the conference was seriously off schedule), they took a break. I was asked to return to the podium afterward, so I was sipping a Diet Coke by myself, staring out of a window, wishing I could be somewhere else, when the brothel association president came up and introduced himself.

He told me he'd been a high school science teacher in California before a friend of his had become the owner of the Chicken Ranch (located in Pahrump—no, that is not a misspelling) and had asked him to become the manager. Because he'd taught science, he said, he understood better what I was saying than did most of the audience. I think he was trying to get me to feel he was sympathetic to my position. But then he said something that immediately and, I think, intentionally put me on guard.

He said that after he moved to Nevada, it took him awhile to become accustomed to the way people did business in the Silver State. Knowing I was a recent move-in, he advised me to slow my approach to policy and take the necessary time to learn how business was done.

For instance, he said, using a wise and conciliatory tone, he knew where I lived, where my kids went to school, where my wife did her grocery shopping, and that it would be for the best if I remembered how much he knew.

He finished by telling me he planned to allow me only a couple of additional questions from the audience and any closing comments I might wish to make before moving the meeting back on to the other topics scheduled.

Less than an hour later, I was in the parking lot looking at my old green Volvo and wondering if it was safe to insert the key and start it since the brothel association president "had my number." But I persuaded myself that if I was ever safe from the brothel association, it would be when starting my car in the parking lot outside their annual meeting.

So I just drove off.

By this time a number of people had warned me about violence as a way of life in Nevada, and particularly inside the brothel community. I don't know how many times I was told that justice in Nevada was a shallow grave in the desert, whatever that was supposed to mean.

I came to the conclusion pretty quickly, though, that I had nothing to worry about, at least not from the bordello businessmen. I ran into them in various odd places, and they were always cordial. One of them came to a chamber orchestra concert at the University of Nevada Reno and sat in front of me and my wife. He had a woman on each arm, and the three of them made a point of trying to make small talk with us during the intermission. My wife found their promiscuous dress and manner to be quite unattractive (she didn't know who they were) and couldn't understand how I came to be so familiar with them. When I explained to her how I knew the man, she found that revelation repulsive.

But there was no hint of danger in any of these chance meetings. It was apparent they considered me an irritant but were not concerned at all about my ability to interrupt their business.

My impression of not being under threat from the brothels was confirmed some months later when a delegation from the brothel association visited Myla Florence, who replaced my boss, Larry Matheis, as health division administrator in 1988.

When they scheduled the meeting, they specifically asked that I be excluded. However, because the air-handling system at the health division building was being serviced, the air ducts in Ms. Florence's office were laid open and, sitting in my own office nearby, I could hear the entire conversation coming through the air diffuser perfectly. The brothel owners had asked for the meeting because they wanted a chance to brief Ms. Florence about how biased and unfair I'd been in releasing information about gonorrhea in the brothels to the press.

In their opinion, I'd acted in that manner not as dispassionately as was expected of a public-health official but had instead been guided by my religious zealotry (that Mormon thing again). They hoped to persuade

Ms. Florence of this point so that she, unlike Larry, would not allow me to send out press releases about STDs in the brothels.

The truth was that even had I continued with press releases about gonorrhea and prostitution, by then no news outlet was taking any interest. It was old news, and no one seemed to care. They (the brothel owners) made it clear they were actively informing everyone who mattered in the state that, as a religious zealot, I was not to be believed when speaking about the business of prostitution. And they believed their campaign had been highly successful. In their opinion, I was more than neutralized and would no longer be a factor with which they concerned themselves. I'm sure they were correct. Only a handful of people were truly interested in the public-health aspect of prostitution.

And it seems only a handful of American citizens ever consider the public-health aspect of American health insurance. Like prostitution, the business interests of American health insurance are in direct conflict with the health interests of those who purchase the service. Prostitution is a purple world where profits are directly related to the frequency of disease-transmitting events. Likewise, health insurance thrives through increasing the likelihood of bad disease or injury outcomes by escaping responsibility for the cost of health care.

Insurers do their best to selectively "cover" only the healthiest people and then deny as many benefits as possible. Claims-processing overhead is commonly as high as 25 percent, meaning that insurance companies use as much as one in four dollars received to find a reason to not pay for care. As mentioned previously, among first-world countries, only in America do we have bake sales to raise the funds needed to care for cancer. And only in America are health-care costs the most common cause of personal bankruptcy, even for those "covered" with insurance. Health insurance is the most wasteful method ever invented to fund health care. Tens of thousands of deaths are caused each year by the health-insurance business model. But for the political clout of the health-insurance industry, surely we Americans would have rid our society of this purple pestilence.

Like the Nevada brothel industry, American health insurers are very good at getting the public to ignore the facts about their business. They're also good at maintaining tight relationships with politicians from both red and blue sides of the aisle.

Thanks to whistleblower Wendell Potter, a former public-relations executive for CIGNA (one of the nation's largest health insurers), we know how health insurers maintain their hold on American politicians. Mr. Potter, who once came to Salt Lake City to speak, said he had an epiphany about how wrong the health-insurance industry was while he was at a health fair held in coal-mining country.

There, he saw thousands of people seeking the medical care being donated by various local providers at the fair. As he became familiar with the people spending hours waiting in lines to get desperately needed care, he realized that the business model of American health insurers had created the catastrophic circumstances of these people's lives. He became ashamed of what he did for a living and soon thereafter left his work. He is now a freelance analyst at the Center for Public Integrity (www.publicintegrity.org), where he posts observations about the politics and economics of health care in America.

Recently, he posted this about health-care markets:

> The reasons Americans tolerate paying so much more for health care than citizens of any other country—and getting less to show for it—is our gullibility. We've been far too willing to believe the self-serving propaganda we've been fed for decades by health insurers and pharmaceutical companies and every other part of the medical-industrial complex, a term *New England Journal of Medicine* editor Arnold Relman coined 35 years ago to describe the uniquely American health-care system. One of the other reasons we tolerate unreasonably high health-care costs is gullibility's close and symbiotic relative: blind adherence to ideology. By this I mean the belief that the free market—the invisible hand Adam Smith wrote about more than two centuries ago and that many

Americans hold as a nonnegotiable tenet of faith—can work as well in health care as it can in other sectors of the economy. While the free market is alive and well in the world's other developed countries, leaders in every one of them, including conservatives, decided years ago that health care is different, that letting the unfettered invisible hand work its magic in health care not only doesn't create the unintended social benefits Smith wrote about, it all too often creates unintended, seemingly intractable, social problems.[6]

Mr. Potter is right. Americans are gullible when it comes to health-care politics and business, just as Nevadans choose to be gullible about prostitution.

Chapter Four

Changing US Health-Care "Business as Usual": A Heavy Political Lift

THE FACT THAT I never had any interest in outlawing prostitution and was not trying to disrupt that business was beside the point for brothel owners. To be sure, I think prostitution is a repugnant practice. But whether it's illegal or, as in some parts of Nevada, not illegal, it does occur. For instance, Clark County, the home county for Las Vegas, where prostitution is illegal, saw a major outbreak of syphilis during my tenure as Nevada's state health officer.

There was an increase in syphilis rates nationwide in the United States beginning in 1986, with several outbreaks in urban areas such as Las Vegas. I remember noting that cases of congenital syphilis (a life-threatening condition in newborns that occurs when pregnant women are infected with syphilis and not promptly treated) suddenly began appearing in Southern Nevada, and I wondered why.

So I posed that question to the director of the Clark County Health District, Dr. Otto Ravenholt. By the late 1980s, Dr. Ravenholt had been the public-health leader in Las Vegas for a quarter century, and he didn't retire until ten years later.

He was generally regarded as an icon in Southern Nevada because he'd found ways to improve sanitation and mental health care in the 1960s. Unquestionably, he was effective, at least early on in his tenure. He's the only local health officer I know of who combined his more than thirty years at the helm of the health department while also serving as the county coroner.

And at various times he was the director of the Nevada State Department of Health and Human Services, the CEO of the county hospital, and a one-time candidate for Congress. A generation older than I am, he was someone I should've been able to look to for help, or at least some mentoring.

He ran the largest health department in the state and, as such, was viewed by members of the legislature from Las Vegas as the leading figure in public health anywhere in Nevada. They always cared more about his opinion than mine, understandably.

But Ravenholt survived the peculiar politics of Las Vegas by knowing everyone without being close to anyone. For instance, he took a public stance opposing the press-release approach to STDs in the brothels, though he privately apologized to me for doing it. He had a way of never really offering a straight opinion about anything. In my view, he could talk more and say less than anyone I've ever known.

So when I approached him about congenital syphilis, he thought my questions were impertinent, and he chose to talk around the question of causation. I think he hoped the problem would go away without any public notice. He generally tried to avoid calling attention to any problem that might reflect badly on Las Vegas and therefore hurt tourism.

But cases of syphilis in Las Vegas doubled—and then doubled again.

An outbreak like that deserved a public-health response, and I was determined there would be one. When Dr. Ravenholt eventually conceded during a telephone call that he didn't know why so many cases were occurring, I took that as an opening to invite an investigation team from the Centers for Disease Control to Las Vegas. Inviting the CDC into the state was one of the few things that was completely on my own prerogative as state health officer.

The CDC never comes into a state uninvited, and they only respond to invitations by the lead state health official. As far as I know, prior to this episode with syphilis in Las Vegas, the CDC had never been invited to Nevada. Of course, when they come, they draw attention to the problem that's occasioned their visit. This was why Dr. Ravenholt was angry with me for having circumvented his stonewalling. Eventually, however, he conceded that it had been the right thing to do. He and I were always uneasy friends.

The two CDC investigators arrived in Nevada shortly after I telephoned their Atlanta office and quickly interviewed a number of cases. Using the information derived through the interviews, they developed a hypothesis that the syphilis outbreak was driven by the then increasingly common practice of exchanging sex for crack cocaine (where was Mrs. Reagan's "Just Say No" when you needed it?).

They proposed to intervene by using food to lure people at high risk for syphilis to strategically placed treatment teams in various neighborhoods throughout the metropolitan area. Once at the treatment location, the at-risk person would get a hamburger only after accepting an injection of penicillin (Thanks, Dr. Fleming).

The CDC investigators also persuaded local law enforcement to inject penicillin into anyone jailed on drug charges. The news media caught onto the CDC investigation and eventually persuaded Dr. Ravenholt to hold a press conference, at which he had a field day showing off the results of the syphilis investigation to the TV cameras. More importantly, the rates of syphilis quickly began to fall to more customary levels.

As a public-health officer, my professional interest lay in attempting to reduce the burden of STDs. I sought to enact, enforce, and fund policies that had the best chance to improve health, no matter what behaviors had placed people at risk for disease.

Because in Nevada business interests always superseded—or should I say trumped—public health, I rarely saw a success like the resolution of the syphilis outbreak. The brothel owners quickly learned that they didn't need to fuss about what I might do or say. They threatened violence, but they really didn't need to do anything about me at all. I was easy to ignore. No one in Nevada seemed to consider how business might improve if better public-health practices prevailed.

Food-borne illnesses, for instance, are common in the United States and elsewhere in the world. At least twice while in a foreign first-world country, I've had an acute gastrointestinal illness I believe to have been caused by contaminated food. In both cases, others of my party who shared the same food were likewise affected, providing the basis for my assertion. I've also had similar episodes of illness while traveling in third-world countries, though most people would find this less surprising.

Outbreaks of *E. coli* or other bacterial-caused food-borne illness in the United States receive a great deal of media attention. Food-borne disease is probably one of the most common types of acute illness, whether in the first or the third world. Yet despite how common these illnesses are, and despite the vast numbers of meals served in buffets and restaurants in Nevada, there had been no outbreaks of food-borne illness reported from Nevada to the CDC for at least ten years prior to my service as state health officer.

Within a few months of my start date in Nevada, I received a telephone call from an unhappy recent visitor to Nevada. She'd traveled with a group of about fifty senior citizens from Northern California to various casinos in Northern Nevada by bus. Somewhere along the route, she said, she and her friends had eaten spoiled food. She knew this because before the end of the trip, virtually everyone had experienced a day of gastrointestinal illness. That bus must've been ripe smelling during the thirty-six-hour period when virtually everyone was vomiting and had diarrhea.

She wanted to know what I was going to do about it.

Truthfully, at the time she made the call, I wasn't sure what I should do about such requests. I had virtually no training in the practicalities of observational epidemiology, which is the science of public-health investigations in the field.

About six months after I arrived in Carson City, I was invited to join a training exercise entitled "Epidemiology in Action" at the headquarters of the Centers for Disease Control in Atlanta, held specifically for state and local health officials. There were about forty people in the group, and it was the first such training held by the CDC for nonemployees.

One of the first learning exercises we carried out as a class was called "Oswego: An Outbreak of Gastrointestinal Illness Following a Church Supper." Beginning with that exercise and continuing on through the various other presentations made by CDC staff during those two weeks in Atlanta, I began to acquire the skills I needed to respond to allegations concerning disease outbreaks.

The Oswego exercise concerned the real-life outbreak of nausea, vomiting, diarrhea, and abdominal pain among the eighty or so participants of a church supper on April 18, 1940, in Lycoming, Oswego County, New York. More than half the people eating supper became sick. They all recovered within about a day of becoming ill. The first cases became ill within just a couple of hours of eating, and no new cases occurred after 2:00 a.m. the next day.

Most of the supper eaters filled out a questionnaire about their health status and the food and drink they'd consumed at the supper. Rates of illness could be calculated among those eating each of the various potluck foods, and the epidemiologic finger was pointed at the vanilla ice cream.

According to the field report included with the exercise, laboratory analysis confirmed that large amounts of *Staphylococcus* (a bacteria) were found in the vanilla ice cream. Nose and throat cultures from the sisters who'd made the ice cream also showed *Staphylococcus* (which meant that my infectious-disease professor at medical school should have added respiratory secretions to urine, feces, and blood/bodily fluids as common sources of purple-world contamination).

What I learned in Atlanta would have provided a framework for responding to the Northern California woman who'd enjoyed a bus ride in Northern Nevada until she and her friends became ill. But there were two obstacles.

First, she'd waited too long to tell me about the incident. When several people with shared food exposure become ill at about the same time, the most logical assumption is that a point or single source of exposure to contaminated food or water has occurred. It's best to collect information from the entire group (both sick and well) as soon as possible so that memories about the symptoms, timing, and food exposure remain fresh.

Second, staying on the bus together for a few days after the illness had started probably allowed for secondary cases to occur (assuming this was an infectious-disease outbreak). Diarrhea and vomiting are wonderful ways to spread infectious agents (purple world). However, I learned that when people become involved with gambling, they lose perspective about little things like diarrhea. Since I wasn't able to trace the source of contamination, I suggested the caller seek medical care if she was still worried about her health, and I left it at that.

Not long after I returned to my office after the two-week training in Atlanta, I received a call from a newspaper reporter in Las Vegas asking me what I planned to do about the dozens of people who were right then being taken by ambulance from a casino hotel on the Las Vegas Strip to local emergency rooms. Apparently, all of these people were sick to their stomachs with diarrhea and vomiting.

I played dumb (not hard to do since I had no information about any such event) and said I'd call him back. Then I called Dr. Ravenholt. He told me he'd heard about the problem and had already been to the casino but felt sure this was a case of people coming to Las Vegas and bringing an illness with them.

I could tell he didn't want me interested in this episode.

But too late. I already was. The few facts I knew after talking with Dr. Ravenholt were startling. More than one hundred people had been transported to the emergency room with abdominal pain, nausea, vomiting, and diarrhea. Some of them had fainted while playing at the slot machines due to dehydration (that is a lot of vomiting and diarrhea).

This had to be a point-source outbreak despite Dr. Ravenholt's wanting it to be otherwise. What was needed was observational epidemiology, and who was better suited to provide it than the Nevada state health officer just recently trained for two weeks at the Centers for Disease Control?

I was sure that whatever had gone wrong in food service (the most likely candidate source for exposure) could be discovered. More importantly, I was sure the gaming industry would want the problem discovered so we all could learn from the failing and improve performance. How could an active public-health investigation be anything other than reassuring to the tourism industry?

How could I be so stupid?

I tried reaching the casino by phone but was not connected to anyone high enough on the food chain (sorry, bad pun again) who felt comfortable talking to me. I left messages. Then I telephoned a health division employee in Las Vegas and asked them to do some snooping around so I could get a few more facts. In this case, my staff member didn't let me down.

The casino was at the time hosting about a thousand people from all over the country who'd come to play in a slot tournament. To participate in a slot tournament, each competitor must find a partner willing to share the entry fee of $1,000 or so. Travel to and from Las Vegas by chartered plane is included in the fee, as is the room shared by each team of two slot tourney players. An opening banquet is provided for all participants. Beginning the following morning, each team is assigned specific slot machines at specific times throughout the day and plays by pulling the handle as fast and often as possible, no coins required.

If your arm tires, your partner pulls for you. Scoring is by some system of point acquisition, and at the end of the tournament (which lasts three or four days) the team with the most points wins a substantial amount of money (maybe $100,000), and a percentage of the entire crowd gets their fees back. The key, of course, is to be at your designated slot machine on time, furiously pulling the handle, motivated by the chance to have all of this Las Vegas fun for free.

Evidently, this particular slot tournament began with a banquet on a Monday night. By Wednesday morning, people were beginning to experience vomiting and diarrhea. Nonetheless, they would appear for their turn at the slot machine and pull the handle for all they were worth. Several of the players fainted right at the slot machine after vomiting, and their partners, rather than attend to the downed and dehydrated person, simply reached over their friends and kept racking up points.

It was, of course, that Wednesday morning I heard from the newspaper reporter and spoke with Dr. Ravenholt, who stopped in at the casino and reported that all of these people from all over the country had somehow all become sick at the same moment with what looked like the same gastrointestinal illness. Another surreal and purple Nevada moment.

I telephoned Dr. Ravenholt again and recited the facts of the event as I had come to understand them. He was not happy that I'd continued looking into the circumstances, but he had to admit that his original hypothesis was highly unlikely. I pointed out that this outbreak deserved an investigation. It was at least as likely as not that the casino was innocent and had merely purchased a spoiled product they'd unknowingly served at the banquet.

Surely, I told him, more information would be better for all parties. He gave me the number of the food-service manager at the casino. Given the emphasis he'd placed on food safety early in his tenure as Clark County health officer, this was the least he could have done.

When I reached him by phone, the casino food-service manager did not wish to discuss the circumstances of the outbreak. He stuck with the line initially authored by Dr. Ravenholt about how unfortunate it was that so many people became ill while they should be enjoying their time in Las Vegas, but they clearly (in his view) had been exposed elsewhere and just happened to be in Nevada when their symptoms developed. He hoped they would all recover.

I asked him for lists of the slot-tournament participants and all the food items served at the banquet. He refused. I pointed out that as food-services manager, he might be buying spoiled product from somewhere else and never know it unless we made the effort to study this outbreak. He refused.

I told him that if an attorney were to ever ask me whether his casino did everything possible to promote the health and safety of its guests, I'd have to answer in the negative. He became angry. And yes, he told me I might have to find another job. By then, these moments began to feel less surreal and more like the reality of my chosen profession. I asked him if I might visit him during my next trip to Las Vegas (which was scheduled for the following week), and he said he would get back to me.

After that rather unsuccessful phone call, I reached out to the gastrointestinal diseases branch at the Centers for Disease Control, where I hoped to get some advice about how best to proceed. I'd met representatives from most of the branches of the CDC (like the ones with the sexually transmitted diseases branch who'd helped me respond to the syphilis outbreak) with offices in Atlanta during my training course. In fact, I'd intentionally walked around the buildings looking for the various programs in order to inform them I was the new state health officer in Nevada and would appreciate their support.

Most of the CDC programs had by then long since been attempting to work directly with state health departments. They all proudly displayed a map of the USA on the doors of their offices with each state colored in according to the level of participation or frequency of the relevant case reports. The state of Nevada was remarkable for consistently being a white field of nonparticipation in the midst of an entire nation colored in to represent a connection to the CDC. Almost none of the programs at the CDC apparently ever managed to have a working relationship with the Nevada Division of Health. I was trying to break the ice. The people I met at the CDC seemed to be enthused to finally have a contact in Nevada.

Unfortunately, on this first attempt to have a phone call with those at the CDC with experience in food-borne disease, I did not reach anyone with whom I'd had contact while in Atlanta. The phone conversation felt rushed, because the official who answered the phone was under a deadline of some sort. When I said that the food-services manager at the subject casino hotel was unwilling to share information, he brushed me off by stating the obvious—that no investigation could occur under those circumstances. He seemed unwilling or unable to advise me about how to proceed.

This was the one interaction with the CDC I found unhelpful during my two-plus years as state health officer. But, to his credit, a few months later, that particular CDC official made a point of reaching out to me and apologizing for not being more responsive.

The Centers for Disease Control is a remarkable public-health gift we Americans make to ourselves and to the world.

A few days later, the food-service manager from the slot-tournament casino called back. The press interest in the outbreak had become intense, and they were not buying the idea that the slot-tournament players all happened to come to Nevada from points throughout the nation already infected. The casino needed to project at least the appearance of concern about this problem, so the food-service manager wanted me to take some steps toward an investigation in order to show the public his employer had some interest in solving or understanding the outbreak.

We agreed to meet when next I traveled to Las Vegas, which was a few days later. By then, of course, all the participants in that particular slot tournament had returned to their homes across the nation, making the job of acquiring data infinitely more difficult. He provided me with a list of all food and beverage items offered and consumed by the tournament players. I fashioned a simple written questionnaire designed to shed light on the various symptoms experienced, including the timing of their onset and the kinds of food and beverages consumed by each individual.

I then arranged to send the questionnaire to all the individuals on the casino registry for the subject slot tournament. The questionnaire was accompanied by a cover letter from the casino asking the recipient to fill out the questionnaire and return it directly to me at the Nevada Health Division, where the data could be kept with the confidentiality allowed by state's statutes governing communicable disease control, such as they were at the time.

As is often the case with outbreak investigations that, like this one, start too late, relatively few of the people invited to complete the questionnaire actually took the time or made the effort to respond. We'd lost our best opportunity to thoroughly investigate this outbreak when the casino rejected my first inquiries out of hand because of their fear of adverse publicity. And then, of course, they suffered from adverse publicity all the same and couldn't defend themselves by showing any effort to respond to the problem. Additionally, because they threw all the leftover food away, we were denied any opportunity to test it for possible contamination at the public-health laboratory.

The casino hotel did not allow me to interview the staff who prepared and served the food. Larry Matheis attempted to induce the governor's office to pressure the casino into cooperation, but the governor was uninterested in disturbing his US Senate campaign by irritating anyone in the gaming industry. We did receive a few dozen responses to our request to the slot-tournament players to fill out a questionnaire, mostly from people who'd become ill. The small size of the sample of people willing to share their personal information with us severely limited the power of the investigation and therefore any ability to draw statistically strong conclusions from review of the data. The preliminary information seemed to link consumption of some Australian lobster with the subsequent development of illness.

A few of those who sent in completed questionnaires also signed release forms allowing me to review the clinical records of their treatment at local Las Vegas hospitals. But I found that they'd received symptomatic care only, and no diagnostic studies, like stool cultures, had been ordered. In summary, we reached a dead end. The press became interested in something else, and so did I. It's impossible to make progress on public-health problems one news cycle at a time. More so when the objective is to change the way we do health-care business. The massive medical industrial complex has momentum funded by the $3 trillion in its revenue stream. Changing the focus of its business model from profits to patients will take an enduring effort by many millions of Americans.

This was not the only time a food-borne outbreak affected dozens of guests at a Las Vegas casino hotel during my time in Nevada. In addition to slot tournaments, which are planned and created by the host facility in order to bring more customers to their doors, many conferences and conventions in Las Vegas occur at the instigation of large groups and corporations.

During my first year as state health officer, a major American fast-food corporation held a special several-day celebration for its top-producing franchise owners from across the nation at a particular casino hotel on the Las Vegas Strip.

If I remember correctly, there were about ten thousand attendees at that event who were treated to open and closing banquets and hours of fun and games in between. Just before these people were scheduled to head to the airport, some of them began experiencing particularly severe bloody diarrhea as well as fever.

This form of abdominal disease is commonly called dysentery. And many more cases erupted after these people arrived at their homes and resumed their work at the fast-food franchises. What was worse for the parent fast-food corporation was that secondary cases began occurring among the customers of the hamburger joints in towns across the country. A vice president of the corporation called me and inquired not so gently concerning what I was planning to do about the problem his company believed started in Nevada.

The first reports of dysentery had, of course, caught my attention. I'd attempted to get the cooperation of the casino hotel staff but had been, as usual, unsuccessful. So I explained to the vice president that my hands were tied by the unwillingness of the Las Vegas facility to provide me with access to the information I needed.

His response was remarkable. He asked me to write down everything I needed for this investigation, including information, personnel, and other resources.

I asked for a complete inventory of the food served during the several-day event and a list of all the hotel staff involved in preparing and serving the food, with a promise of access to interview them if necessary.

I required a list of the franchise participants, all ten thousand of them. I indicated that two CDC EIS (Epidemic Intelligence Service) officers, with whatever equipment they stipulated, would be needed to organize and process the data collection. And I threw in that having an office available in Las Vegas near the casino hotel would be ideal.

The vice president promised that everything would be ready by the next day. And it was. He himself arrived in Las Vegas to oversee the implementation of the investigation. He announced that he'd asked the CDC for information about how to sanitize every fast-food franchise facility located near participants in the recently concluded corporate celebration. Once he had the CDC directive regarding the sanitizing of the restaurants, he supervised the task of closing and cleaning the thousands of affected stores nationwide during the next seventy-two hours.

And the casino-hotel staff fell all over themselves to please him. The bacterial agent causing the dysentery was identified by laboratory tests done in Atlanta by the CDC. All of the ill people were appropriately treated. People who had not become ill were taken off duty until the possible incubation period had passed and they no longer represented a risk to the public.

Most compelling was the insistence by the fast-food corporation that everything done should be clearly documented and explained to the public. Unlike the typical Nevada approach, this company believed the public would understand and appreciate that bad things happen to good, well-meaning people. Further, they believed the public would applaud a well-executed response to the crisis and not take their business elsewhere.

Imagine that: public health and good business can coexist, with both thriving.

Over the years I've spent in public health, particularly when advocating for health-system reform, I've repeatedly heard from would-be critics that we Americans must downsize our expectations. Such criticism is usually framed as pragmatism, like "Don't let the perfect get in the way of the good" or "A half loaf is better than none." Good public-health practice is, however, both pragmatic and all-or-nothing. When we invoke our best public-health science in order to make the best public-health policy and deliver the optimum public-health practice, we are doing what is always pragmatic, which is protecting our nation's greatest asset: the health of our citizens. No one effectively attacks the purple world with rose-colored glasses. I eschew idealism. But there's nothing to be gained by doing only what is politically expedient and calling the effort good. Every excess illness, injury, or death that could have been prevented is a drain on American productivity. In our health system, half-loaf measures like Obamacare and its mean-spirited corollary, Trumpcare, are massively expensive and still leave millions of us without an effective chance to live productively and realize the American promise to pursue life, liberty, and happiness.

Winston Churchill was supposed to have said that Americans would always do the right thing—after they'd tried every other alternative.

Surely we've given the misguided, self-serving political interests every opportunity to help us really reform American health-care delivery. Now would be a good time for us to begin choosing a better way to conduct health-care business. If we fail to find a way to rid ourselves of business as usual in American health care, we'll go on wasting a trillion dollars a year and bankrupting our nation. Virtually all the projected federal budget deficit throughout the working lives of my children's generation is due to the incredible cost of health care.

What I call waste, of course, is known to health-care corporations as profit. They'll defend their profits politically with all the force their vast sums of money can apply. Jon Huntsman Jr. (R-UT), when in the first year of his first term as governor, actually had his staff work on a modest piece of legislation I suggested to him. There is in Utah (uniquely, I believe) a nonprofit, private trust fund—the Public Employees Health Plan (PEHP)—that pays for the health-care benefit given to many public employees who work for state and local governments. PEHP is very efficient, with an overhead 75 percent less than the larger, private health insurers in Utah. I proposed that the enabling statutes that created PEHP be altered such that PEHP could sell its efficient health benefit to private citizens. This would have been a very small step in the right direction.

But the health-insurance industry vigorously opposed this as if their very existence was being threatened. During the session that bill was introduced, I attempted to persuade a number of legislators to vote for its passage. I never spoke to any legislator without having an insurance lobbyist corner him or her within a few steps of leaving the conversation with me. The bill sponsor found himself at odds with a powerful lobby. Other unrelated bills he was sponsoring were held up and threatened. He eventually caved to the pressure.

Make no mistake, any real change in US health policy is going to require heavy political lifting. In fact, it will only happen when politicians learn by sad experience that the American public will kick them out of office if they pander to the health-care corporate interests at the expense of good patient care.

The high cost and poor health outcomes of the American way of doing health care are an economic drag on the American way of life. Ridding our nation of the trillion-dollar annual waste due to poor-quality care (inappropriate care, patient injury, and failing to deliver best clinical care consistently) and inefficient financing of health care would stimulate economic growth beyond just the trillion dollars saved.

People would be healthier. And they would be freer to choose a more entrepreneurial career path. Real health-system reform would virtually eliminate the federal deficit over the next several decades, completely remaking our opportunities for real tax reform. American businesses, after decades of carrying ridiculous health-benefit costs, would rapidly become much more competitive in a global economy. Government funds now destined for health-care programs could be used to inject new life into another major public enterprise: education. Revitalizing American education would, over time, create a more tech-savvy American populace, better able to grow the American economy.

Health-system reform is the signal domestic issue in America. We either get this right, as Winston Churchill says we will, or we face a future of economic decline, perhaps into second-world status. I'm not an economist, but I am certain the current business practices of American health care are not sustainable. We simply can't afford to have relentless growth in the share of our gross domestic product going to health care. Former secretary of Health and Human Services Michael Leavitt has said that there is no place on the world's leaderboard for a nation spending 25 percent of its GDP on health care. The United States either reforms health-care delivery or ceases to be a world leader.

Chapter Five

The Power of Constitutional Federalism and Perverse Incentives in US Health Care

During the summer of 1989, the Rainbow Family held their annual prayer for peace celebration in the Jarbidge Wilderness north of Elko, Nevada. This was to be the twentieth annual celebration, a tradition that allegedly has its roots at the rock concert held at Woodstock, New York, in the 1960s.

According to those involved, these events are supposed to be anarchic, meaning no one is in charge. They just happen. Someone finds the location, someone else publicizes it, and a number of people come early to set up a "seed" camp to get things started. People bring food, or medical supplies, or cooking utensils, or whatever they have and can share. Supposedly everything always turns out perfectly well, every year.

Except for 1987, when shigellosis (a type of dysentery) hit the Rainbow Family gathering in North Carolina and followed many of them home afterward, where many dozens of secondary cases began to spread. Evidently, anarchy can mean that some people poop where other people are trying to find drinking water (remember the purple world?). Diarrhea makes this problem, of course, much worse, especially where hand-washing facilities are rare, even in food-preparation areas. Once Nevada became the destination for the Rainbow Family in 1989, I began to hear from a number of federal officials warning me that Nevada could be the next national epicenter for dysentery if I didn't do something about it.

Fortunately, Myla Florence was supportive of the use of health division time and resources in an effort to reduce the risk of water-borne disease at the Rainbow Camp. I discovered where to contact some of the non-leaders of the movement, with whom I had pointed conversations about the need for sanitation—and not just if it happened to occur through the goodwill and voluntarism of family members. I referred them to the army field manual and asked them to be sure to construct latrines according to military specifications. Soap for hand-washing was to be mandatory at every food-preparation area. Food was to be prepared and handled according to army standards. Myla arranged to have one of the health division inspectors on-site throughout the heavily populated days of the camp (approximately one week before and one week after July 4) so that he could verify compliance or let us know in a timely fashion if problems occurred. Myla and I personally traveled to the camp for a day late in June, which was quite a safari.

We arrived the night before in Elko, arose at 4:00 a.m. the next morning, and took a four-hour drive north. We then hiked five miles into the wilderness, where we began encountering the crowd, estimated that year at something just less than ten thousand. They were located in camps stretching about a mile along a beautiful mountain stream. Clothes were optional for the Rainbows, as was following local laws and ordinances.

One story that received some circulation at the time concerned a Rainbow fellow who allegedly entered a grocery store, went to the bread section, took two slices from a loaf, took the slices to the deli and helped himself to two slices of baloney from a package, placed these on the bread, then went to the condiment aisle and opened and used a jar of mayonnaise, then left the store munching a sandwich.

Fortunately, there was a good deal of forbearance among the law-enforcement officers, otherwise there could have been a few full jails in Elko. Bathing was particularly optional; I remember walking into a wall of body odor before discovering the source of the smell (two naked people) coming over a rise along the trail.

But the hand soap was visible in every kitchen, and the latrines were dug per army protocol. Water was drawn upstream from camp, and no one went home sick. It was a memorable day. Myla and I ate the food we brought with us for lunch before heading back along the five-mile trail and thence to Elko's small airport and home. No outbreak of shigellosis occurred while the Rainbow Family enjoyed their anarchic holiday. Likewise, the American health-care system can remain in private hands, and local, even as needed discipline is imposed upon it by a combination of federal and state regulation, with the states taking the lead while getting federal backing, not unlike the time-honored practice of state health agencies taking the lead in delivering public-health services but always able to get assistance from the Centers for Disease Control.

One other food-borne outbreak, however, that occurred during my tenure as state health officer is worth mentioning. Until about the year 2000, no vaccine for hepatitis A was widely available. During the second half of the twentieth century, there were twenty- to sixty-thousand cases of this viral disease per year in the USA. Nationwide, slowly evolving epidemic cycles were observed with peaks in 1961, 1971, and 1989.

Early in 1989, there was a distinct surge in hepatitis A in Carson City, the capital of Nevada. Hepatitis A spreads from person to person via the previously described fecal-oral route—disgusting and quite common—of course (purple world, again).

So we took the increase in case counts seriously and began contacting the people who suffered the disease to ask them about the food and water sources. Unlike dysentery, hepatitis A has an incubation period of up to two months, averaging about one month. So, if there were to be a point source, naturally it would have been something that occurred a month or so before the symptoms became obvious. Further, asymptomatic infections and/or mild illness can be common, meaning that much of the burden of infection can be entirely undetected in a community.

This means an investigation can't target a specific list of foods served during a distinct time interval, at least initially. One of the curious things noted after interviewing about a dozen patients who had had hepatitis A during early 1989 in Carson City was that all of these people were employees of the state of Nevada, though not from a single state agency.

This, of course, drew our attention to the food sources commonly available to state employees, and that quickly led us to the vending machines in every state building, all of which were serviced by a single proprietor. Most of the items sold in these vending machines were pre-packaged snacks from nationally known brands. It seemed unlikely that if hygiene practices were failing for these national companies, the cases would only show up in Carson City government buildings. Therefore, we focused our attention on the products of local origin, mostly sandwiches.

The vending-machine sandwiches were all made by one small delicatessen in Carson City. We sent a sanitarian to the deli to take a quick look at the facility. His report was disgusting. The deli had no sink other than in the one bathroom on-site, and that sink was not operational. The bathroom itself was disgustingly dirty, with a filthy toilet and floor (I leave that purple world to the reader's imagination). Each employee, present and former, was contacted and interviewed. This was a small list of people because the deli principally made sandwiches for vending machines. Very few customers were actually served on-site (not surprising, given the uninviting milieu).

One of the employees had actually developed hepatitis A with jaundice during the preceding fall (1988), roughly two incubation periods back in time before the current outbreak in Carson City began. I developed the hypothesis that this previous employee who developed hepatitis had probably passed the disease to a coworker who, though remaining asymptomatic him or herself, nonetheless passed the virus on to vending-machine buyers some two months later. An alternative hypothesis would have been that a supplier of sandwich makings was the source of the contamination.

The outbreak drew attention from the Northern Nevada media. I remember arriving by plane at the Reno airport during the time of this outbreak investigation and encountering several TV camera crews with their bright lights just inside the terminal. There were some local personal-injury attorneys who thought they might be able to recruit a remunerative case or two as well. Ultimately, as always happens, interest waned as the news cycle moved on. I chose to leave the source of the outbreak open-ended in the final report, having been unable to completely rule out the possibility of a contaminated food source upstream from the deli. The deli itself lost its vending contract and closed permanently, which, in any case, clearly improved food safety in Carson City for the general public.

But the attention to hepatitis A in Northern Nevada in early 1989 had an interesting follow-up story. One of the people with hepatitis A who'd been contacted by health-department staff turned out to be an employee of a local restaurant and not a state government agency. This restaurant was located directly across the street from the Nevada legislature, which was in session in early 1989.

Because of its proximity to the state capitol, this restaurant was commonly frequented at lunch by members of the legislature and their usual cadre of suitors for legislative favor. It seemed reasonable to me to send a sanitarian to the restaurant to inquire about food-handling practices, given that one of their servers had just been identified as a case of hepatitis A. What we found were some important variations in hygienic practice.

For instance, not uncommonly at this restaurant, servers would toss salads with their bare hands. If the server with hepatitis A had handled salad with bare hands during the days prior to the onset of his symptoms (and he would not say one way or the other), and if he had possibly failed to adequately wash his hands on one or more of those days (which he vehemently denied, but then, who would admit to failing to wash?), it was possible that some of the customers who'd eaten those salads were exposed to and incubating hepatitis A.

Back in 1989, before the advent of a vaccine, the standard practice was to offer those exposed to hepatitis A a passive immunization with an intramuscular injection of immune globulin. Consequently, we made the decision to offer immune-globulin injections to any patron of the restaurant during the appropriate exposure time frame and sent out a press release to that effect. Members of the Nevada legislature asked for the privilege of having public-health nurses come to their building for a special clinic so that they could more efficiently, conveniently, and privately take advantage of the offer of immune-globulin injections.

Their request was, of course, granted, but I remember noting the irony that they had just previously denied funding for a similar request for Nevada State employees who may have been exposed to contaminated sandwiches. Rank has its privileges. The public-health nurses, noting the importance of distinguishing rank, told me they'd reserved their larger gauge needles for the injection clinic held at the Nevada legislature.

All attempts to achieve real health-system reform are filtered through this same legislative sieve. State and federal legislators are perhaps the only job category with 100-percent well-funded health financing. None of the legislators anywhere in the country, as they contemplate health-system reform measures, can understand what it feels like to have limited or no financing for needed health care. In self-serving fashion, they assure them-selves an optimal health-insurance package, often on a lifetime basis, even after leaving office. Refusing to reelect these politicians is far better than a large-gauge needle to get them to attend to the health-care needs of the average citizen. Until elected leaders are routinely thrown out of office for failing to reform our health-care system, they will not make the needed changes. They will continue to tell us what we want to hear while taking political donations from the medical industrial complex. They will con-tinue to allow health-care corporate lobbyists to write legislation and rules and even fashion budgets, giving away the public's interests and tax money. If you want this to stop, you must do the necessary political heavy lifting— you must repeatedly throw people out of office until they get the message.

Another business interest versus public-health episode that occurred during the 1989 session of the Nevada legislature concerned vaccine-preventable disease. The gaming industry proposed a change in the requirements for registering children in day-care centers, specifically allowing for an absence of immunization documentation. Dr. Ravenholt actually weighed in on the side of the gaming-industry proposal, stating that this would not have any ramifications for public-health practice.

I disagreed. My experience with investigating vaccine-preventable disease problems was limited, but there had been a case of measles in a school located south of Carson City. The index case had not been age-appropriately vaccinated and had been on an international trip with fam-ily. She came down with measles symptoms not long after returning to the United States.

There was an increase in measles in the United States during 1989–91, with sustained outbreaks occurring in school populations. As often occurred in vaccine-preventable outbreaks, there were secondary cases at the Northern Nevada school, and the public-health nurses found the school's immunization records not nearly complete. This contributed to the difficult process of containing public anxiety about the outbreak while still assuring everyone that every child was appropriately immunized. I couldn't imagine why the public-health community, including Dr. Ravenholt, would preemptively give up on requiring day-care centers to insist on vaccine records upon registration of a child.

Of course, during the intervening decades since my tenure as Nevada state health officer, many Americans have increasingly sought to avoid vaccinating their children. This is leading to measles transmission through casual contact in public venues such as Disneyland, with many dozens of cases occurring over wide geographic areas. I suppose the remarkable success of immunization programs worldwide has led some to believe that the world really is not very purple after all. We've forgotten that the generation who lived through the Great Depression and won World War II also won the war against polio.

I had a classmate during my school years who suffered from polio as a child, but none of my children ever had that experience. Perhaps that is the reason my children's generation, now the parents of America's children, sees no need for the polio vaccine.

But the gaming industry had a business need. They'd begun advertising to broaden the appeal of gambling from swinging singles to families. Increasingly, there were attractions added to casino hotels that would appeal to children. Nevertheless, when it came time for the parents to gamble, the children needed to be somewhere else and not amongst the slot machines or gaming tables. Leaving young children unattended in a hotel room would not appeal to many parents (hopefully), so day-care (or should we say "anytime day-or-night-"care) facilities were being added to the amenities.

The problem was that most parents failed to bring the family's immunization records on their trip to Las Vegas. The solution was simple, at least from the perspective of the gaming industry. Stop requiring the parents to bring the documents. It wasn't difficult for the industry to get a legislative sponsor. The bill passed easily, and I put up little resistance. Now, as vaccine-preventable disease is rising in incidence in the United States, it is notable that pockets of both conservatives and liberals are ignoring the call to immunize. Conservatives who refuse vaccines do so, often, out of mistaken loyalty to the principle of autonomy over doing what is best for their children. Liberals who opt out of vaccines even though they generally fashion policy from scientific fact are failing to recognize the science behind immunization practices. Whether due to misplaced values or misinformed science, parents who fail to protect their offspring are deliberately painting a more purple world for their children. Health-system reform fails, likewise, because conservatives confuse their values and liberals lose their grip on the facts.

I wondered whether I should ever try to resist the gaming industry in Nevada. This was the industry that managed to have the case law of Nevada read that no casino employee could acquire lung cancer or any lung disease from secondhand smoke at the workplace, or at least not be compensated for it.

In 1992, not long after I left Nevada, a lifelong nonsmoking casino worker filed a worker's compensation case alleging that exposure to secondhand tobacco smoke at work was the cause of his lung disease. In fact, there is no doubt that workers in casinos have high exposures to secondhand tobacco smoke.

Secondhand-smoke exposure levels in casinos can be two to eighteen times higher than in offices, and 1.5 to twelve times higher than in restaurants. In the 1992 case, a majority of justices on the Nevada Supreme Court concluded that secondhand-smoke-related illnesses aren't covered by the state's workers compensation law because they aren't considered an occupational disease specific to the casino industry the way black-lung disease is inextricably linked with coal mining.

In fact, one of the justices said that in spite of the frequent presence of smoke in casinos and the associated health risks, Nevada's worker's compensation system could go bankrupt if workers were entitled to financial compensation for smoke-related problems. Clearly, the business interests of Nevada's gaming industry far outweighed any value that might be placed on human life.

When it comes to discussing policies that affect the gaming industry in Nevada, public health never gets dealt a hand. It's not even allowed into the smoke-filled back room. Resistance to bad public-health policy is futile if it happens to be supported by gaming in Nevada. The purple world exists for a reason. What makes good business sense even though it neither conforms to the values of most Americans nor squares with the facts of clinical science can be forced upon the gullible American public if supported with all the power politics of the medical industrial complex.

The gaming industry was not alone in simply not caring about what the public-health impact of their proposals or practices might be. Most businesses, and many individuals, simply assumed the health division was irrelevant, and didn't bother to ask for our input.

There was an underlying assumption that public health, as part of the government, was incompetent and likely to be in the way, and usually for no good reason. I once spoke with a citizen who was unwilling to meet the specifications in public-health regulations for digging a well on his private property. He called to complain to me after failing to persuade the health division staff whose job it was to review well-construction plans for compliance with the regulations passed by the Nevada Board of Health. He began the conversation by stating that undoubtedly I was an incompetent physician because if I had any ability at all, I'd be practicing in the private sector rather than slopping at the public trough. Ironically, these same dismissive attitudes were articulated by those who, having found that their private well had been contaminated somehow, would rail against me for failing to prevent that contamination. This antigovernment sentiment needs to be tempered with the realization that bad bureaucracies exist in the private sector as well. Further, failing public agencies can be held accountable by an electorate, assuming voter willingness to do the hard work of making informed choices at the ballot box. Corporate bureaucracies do not have public accountability, and their officers are never sworn to assure the public's pursuit of life, liberty, and happiness.

Some restaurants in very small, rural Nevada communities would be visited for inspection infrequently because the health division staff had offices many miles distant. In such circumstances, the health inspector would spend an entire day visiting one town with maybe two restaurants due to the travel time involved. Inevitably, however, they would only be able to inspect one of the restaurants because the restaurant not visited first would hear that the official was in town and simply close until he left.

The health division section responsible for inspecting long-term care facilities encountered similar hostility in rural Nevada.

During the inspection of a nursing home located in Elko, the health division team leader, a retired surgeon, contacted me, indicating that nearly all of the staff employed at the facility had converted their tuberculosis (TB) skin test to positive during the interval since the previous inspection. He wanted to inquire with me whether that finding was anything to be concerned about. The answer seemed more than obvious to me. Until proven otherwise, recent TB skin test conversions from negative (unlikely to have been infected with *tubercle bacillus*, the organism which causes tuberculosis) to positive (probably infected with *tubercle bacillus* but likely not diseased in the absence of symptoms) in a group of employees at a nursing home very probably meant that an active case of pulmonary tuberculosis was in the facility and through coughing was exposing the staff.

Given that most of the patients in the nursing home were elderly, it seemed likely that this undiagnosed active case of TB would be one of the patients. The team leader thanked me for my response and told me that his group did not have the expertise to search the facility for the active case.

The Nevada AIDS Task Force was still preparing for the 1989 legislative session but had already made some recommendations, among which was the creation of an entirely new position within the health division: state epidemiologist.

So Larry Matheis and I hired the first state epidemiologist ever employed by Nevada, Debra Brus, a young veterinarian enthused about the possibilities of making a difference in this new capacity (sound familiar?). And she was willing to put up with the remarkably low salary we had available to pay her (yes, very familiar), since the AIDS Task Force had no authority to generate the needed funds for the position. We promised to help her get a master's degree in public health through an off-campus program. But I immediately deployed her in Elko to search for the active case of TB.

And she found it not among the patients but among the nursing-home staff. The director of nutrition had been treated for tuberculosis as a youngster and had had no problems for decades. However, recently she'd begun having issues with arthritis and had been placed on corticosteroid treatments by her local physician.

This treatment helped her joint pain immensely, apparently, and perhaps that was why she ignored the onset of nocturnal fevers and cough. She was probably ill and contagious with TB for weeks before we happened to have a scheduled nursing-home review, which occasioned the discovery of her disease. People in the nursing home, both staff and patients, considered her the unofficial matron of the place and sought her time and attention often. She had a small office where she would entertain whoever needed solace, an ideal situation for the inadvertent passage of an infective dose of TB containing respiratory droplets (more ways the world can be purple).

In light of Dr. Brus's discovery, the Nevada Health Division officially mandated that the nursing home arrange for several things to occur immediately. First, the nutritionist who had active TB would be placed on leave and receive proper treatment. Second, every patient and staff member would be screened for active tuberculosis. And, third, all persons who had a documented conversion of their TB skin test from negative to positive would receive prophylactic treatment as per the guidance of the American Thoracic Society, the lead resource of widely accepted protocols for handling tuberculosis in the United States. The threat to the nursing home was that we would not give them a passing grade on their facility inspection without compliance.

Unfortunately, the nursing home did not care to comply. They insisted that the Nevada Health Division had no authority in either statute or regulation to mandate these responses to this case. If I remember correctly, the nursing home simply fired the nutritionist and went on with the pretense of business as usual. In essence, they dared us to do anything about it.

They went further. The Nursing Home Association defended the Elko facility and lobbied the governor, asking him to get the health division out of the way. The written media began paying attention to the case, pressing the governor's office for a statement about whether he would back the health division. As I've already noted, the governor was in a campaign for the US Senate seat and chose to avoid antagonizing any possible allies, especially one that, like the Nursing Home Association, could turn into a political enemy. So he made a statement to the effect that the health division had botched the inspection and therefore the nursing home should be exonerated.

When a newspaper reporter caught up with Dr. Brus and gave her a chance to respond, she said that the governor's statement was grade-D baloney. Larry Matheis was personally chastised by Governor Bryan for that miscue by Debra. I think this episode, more than anything else, made Larry's decision soon thereafter to leave the health division easy for him.

Larry Matheis proposed what seemed like a reasonable solution to our stalemate with the nursing home. He asked me to write emergency regulations covering the discovery of a case of infectious disease in a nursing home. This would grant the state health officer authority to mandate appropriate responses to such a threat.

The monthly state board of health meeting was scheduled within a few days of this impasse with the nursing home. Larry served as the (nonvoting) secretary to the board, and I was its principle source of public-health data and scientific information, attending every meeting and testifying often. We both felt the board members would be sympathetic to the need for a vigorous response to communicable disease threats in nursing homes.

We were wrong. The board refused to pass the emergency regulations. They indicated they might well vote in favor of the regulations after they jumped through the usual hoops (public hearings all over the state, responses to all comments to the proposed regulations, etc.) but that nothing in the current case in Elko required urgent expansion of the authority of the state health officer.

Given the chairman's response to gonorrhea, perhaps I should've anticipated this rejection of a reasonable request. In any case, the Elko nursing-home administration was feeling quite smug. I did start the process of passing the regulations but knew the process was time-consuming. The health division also organized a one-day education seminar on communicable diseases in nursing homes, which we offered in several different venues across the state.

There was a final chapter to this incident, however. Not long after losing the vote on emergency regulations at the state board of health meeting, I received a call from the regional administrator of the US Department of Health and Human Services in San Francisco. He asked me about the situation in Elko, which I outlined for him. The refusal of the nursing-home administration to comply with the health division's eminently reasonable mandates angered him. He told me he was responsible for the payment of the federal portion of the Medicaid bills from nursing homes in Nevada. Further, he indicated that none of the Elko nursing-home bills would be paid until he had received in writing a statement from me that the administration in that facility was in full compliance with our mandates, whether official regulations existed or not.

A few days after that phone call, the Elko nursing-home administrator was on the phone with me asking for information about what he needed to do to make the situation right. For some reason, the Nursing Home Association never reported that to the press or to Governor Bryan. This episode illustrates best how constitutional federalism can work in the US health-care system. State governments are close to the people and should know best what services are needed. In the event, however, that state or local government can't or won't deliver the needed services, the federal government can provide a powerful inducement or requirement for better outcomes. In America, there are eighty thousand different governmental entities, from the federal level to the local sewer district. We actually don't hate government here, we use it to do those things that require all of us to work together for our collective good.

One would think that a nursing home should, perhaps more readily than any business, esteem the needs of its helpless patients higher than its own self-interest. But that's not the case in the United States. Nursing homes are principally for-profit. The owners of these facilities expect to maximize their investment in the enterprise. They hire directors of these institutions who have one fiduciary duty only: make as much money as possible for the investors. I suppose the blatant power play by the gaming industry to create the political fantasy that secondhand smoke in a casino doesn't cause occupational lung cancer is business as usual and to be expected. But "business as usual" in American health-care institutions is no less blatantly self-serving and equally dangerous to life and health, especially to those among us who most need help: patients.

American patients are dying by the tens of thousands per year due to preventable injuries sustained in hospitals. As mentioned, it is the fifth leading cause of death in the United States. It's time you and every other American citizen begin caring about the perverse incentives inherently part of business as usual in American health care. *Remember: we do not have the world's best health-care system, we have the world's most profitable health-care system.*

Chapter Six

Rabies at the Laundry—
Bipartisan Failure in Health Policy

THE PERSON-TO-PERSON SPREAD of disease was not the only kind of communicable disease Nevada Public Health had to contend with. Plague continues to be a threat throughout the American West, with a reservoir in ground squirrels. Of course, it's not the squirrels that are a threat to humans but the fleas on the squirrels, which fleas are infected with *Yersinia pestis,* the plague Bacillus, and which may search for a blood meal from a passing human.

Surveillance of rodents and their fleas was a constant requirement in Nevada, particularly in popular camping or hiking areas or in the suburbs where wild rodents coexisted with humans in their neighborhoods. Where plague was found among rodents and/or their fleas, health department posters were tacked to surrounding telephone poles and trees, informing the public to keep their distance from rodent colonies and reminding them not handle the dead animals.

I lived with my family in a suburb south of Reno where plague posters were commonly on display. I taught my boys to stay clear of the marmots that inhabited the pasture across the street from our house. Whenever one of the marmots died (usually a casualty on the road caused by a passing car), I would bury the body to keep my kids from getting too close. We had a case or two of the plague in Nevada during my time at the State Health Office, including a Washoe County Health Department employee who put himself in harm's way while dusting an area to suppress flea populations.

Most of the public-health time and effort associated with zoonotic disease prevention, however, is spent on rabies. It is a fearful disease characterized by apprehension, fever, headache, and malaise at first and evolving to paralysis and muscle spasms, and almost uniformly to the demise of the patient. There are around forty thousand human rabies deaths per year worldwide, but most of these are in third-world countries that have little control over domestic animals, particularly dogs. These feral animals are the reservoir for this deadly disease.

In the United States from 1980 to 1997, only thirty-six human rabies deaths were recorded. There were no human rabies cases in Nevada during my tenure, though I spent a lot of time answering questions about whether various people with animal bites should be vaccinated for rabies. In Nevada, as in much of the western United States, the principle animal reservoir for rabies was the insectivorous bat. One would think that humans rarely encounter bats, but that wasn't my experience as a public-health officer.

For instance, I received a frantic phone call from the administrator of a small hospital in Winnemucca, Nevada, asking what should be done about bats flying throughout his facility. Winnemucca is a town of a few thousand people located along I-80 between Reno and Salt Lake City.

At the time I was working in Nevada, road signs along the freeway nearby trying to attract drivers into this enterprising town read "Winnemucca: 6 billion people have never been here!"

The Winnemucca hospital was an old county building with thick walls in which a colony of bats had long been prospering. For reasons not known to me, after years of tolerating the colony, someone decided the bats must be eliminated, so all of the various access points used by the bats were identified and sealed off. Unfortunately, this well-meaning person chose to seal these access points during the day, when the bats were roosting in the wall. After sunset, when the bats were ready to feed, they found the usual exits closed, and as hunger increased in the colony, a frantic effort to exit ensued.

Eventually the bats found a way out of the wall, but instead of emerging on the outside of the building, they emerged inside. Of course, the patients had to be evacuated until the building could be rid of the bats and sanitized. But this evacuation required moving the patients many miles away to several nearby towns in order to find sufficient bed space to accommodate them.

More commonly than from hospitals, I received calls about managing bat populations from casino hotels in Reno. Bat colonies roosted under highway bridges around the Truckee Meadows and usually found ample opportunities to feed on insects attracted to the bright beams lighting up the hotel buildings around town.

In the largest of these casino hotels one morning, a maid actually found a dead bat in the bedding. The occupant of the previous night had checked out and not reported the bat to the hotel desk clerk. Presumably he was unaware of the bat, which had gotten into the room through an open window.

The maid reported the bat to her supervisor, and eventually the bat was taken to the state laboratory for testing and was found to be rabid. At that point, I received a phone call from the laboratory director indicating that there had been possible human contact with a rabid animal.

A telephone call to the hotel, now a couple of days after the discovery of the bat, revealed that the room occupant was a native of Germany, and I was given his address in Europe. I had served a two-year proselyting mission in German-speaking Europe (Austria) just over a decade before my appointment to serve in Nevada, so with my German language skills, I decided to attempt by telephone to locate a local health department in the hometown of the possibly rabies-exposed hotel visitor.

I believed the best outcome in this case was for a local public-health official to first understand the situation (we found a dead, rabid bat in this man's sheets) and then offer the appropriate public-health services to him according to German laws and customs, whatever those might be. I telephoned the Centers for Disease Control for information about how to make contact with German public-health authorities. They provided some useful ideas about how to begin the search, and after a few other phone calls, I actually did speak with someone in the hotel patron's hometown.

I conveyed the message about the rabid bat (*die Pfledermaus*) to the German public-health authority and left the matter in his hands. The message got through at least to some extent because I later received a phone call from a reporter in Germany who was writing a story for a newspaper about this event.

But that episode was easy compared to what happened at the International Bar in Austin, Nevada. Located on Highway 50 (the Loneliest Highway in America) in the heart of Nevada, the town of Austin is a very small place that has no business naming any business there "international."

Not far from town, apparently, there was a gold mine that provided employment for some of the town's male citizens. Two of these miners finished their shift one Friday evening and headed to the parking lot, where one of them had parked his pickup, ready for a night of partying.

They had stashed some beer in the truck so they could begin drinking as soon as the shift ended, which they did. One of the two men noticed a dead bat lying next to the truck and, for reasons unknown, picked the bat up and tossed it into the bed of the truck before they drove off. I don't know what they did for the next several hours. Neither of them could remember anything at all from the entire evening. However, eyewitnesses, including the barkeep at the International Bar, told me what happened later in the evening when these two very drunk miners came into that establishment.

One of the two had the dead bat stuck in his shirt pocket as they walked up to the bar. They ordered one drink each and a third that was evidently intended for the bat. Having had the drinks placed on the bar in front of them, the man with the bat in his shirt took the bat out and helped it to "taste" the whiskey, dipping its head into the shot glass. He then tied the bat onto his wrist with some string and began flying the bat around the room, zooming over other patrons and making a general nuisance of himself and the dead animal.

Eventually, the bat began dive-bombing into its own whiskey, which of course, spilled all over the bar. Thirsty (at least according to the miners who were serving as very loud spokesmen for the dead animal), apparently the bat then went after other people's drinks, which caused a great deal of commotion. People took great exception to having a bat invade their alcoholic beverages. Because of their fellow patrons' distress, the miners then felt the need to chastise the bat for his misbehavior. As punishment, one of the miners untied the bat from his wrist with his teeth and then held the creature in his mouth with his teeth and shook the animal from side to side.

The eyewitnesses were stunned by this turn of events, because, when interviewed later, none of them could recall whether only one of the miners had held the bat in his teeth or whether they had taken turns punishing the bat. The drunken behavior lasted quite some time, but eventually the two men lost interest in the bat, left it languishing on the bar, and departed for parts unknown. The barkeeper gingerly slid the bat off the bar with some kind of implement and into the garbage.

Later, the barkeeper told a county sheriff's deputy about the incident when the lawman stopped in for some coffee in the middle of the night. The deputy asked if the dead bat was still within reach because he had seen a Nevada Health Division poster advising that any dead bat in direct contact with humans should be sent to the state laboratory for rabies testing. The barkeeper fished the dead animal out of the trash can and packaged it up for the deputy, who set off on his solitary rounds for the night.

During the night, law enforcement officers arranged to rendezvous with each other all along Highway 50 heading west from Austin, passing the dead bat from one county to the next, until a highway patrolman brought the bat to the state laboratory in Reno sometime over the weekend. A couple of days later, as I remember, just prior to the Thanksgiving weekend, I first received word about this incident by way of a telephone call from the laboratory director informing me that a rabid bat had been in direct contact with humans.

The laboratory director gave me the phone number of the highway patrolman who'd been the final carrier of the carcass, and from him I eventually tracked the bat back to the International Bar.

I telephoned the bar and spoke with the barkeeper, who gave me the history, recounted above, of the antics of the two patrons inside his establishment. He asked around at the bar and was able to supply the names of the two miners. Eventually, I was able to speak to them by telephone as well, though the only thing they remembered at all from the evening in question was initially finding and keeping the bat.

The question I felt compelled to answer was whether the exposure to the bat, now known to be rabid, was sufficient to cause a necessity for immunization. The two men themselves were not particularly interested in the multiple injections and expense required to vaccinate them against this terrible disease. But still, I didn't wish to dismiss the possibility of rabies exposure lightly. It would've been poor public-health practice to have known about this incident, done nothing, and then found that one or both of the miners had died of rabies.

I called the rabies program at the Centers for Disease Control to get their opinion. It was after hours in Atlanta by the time I tried reaching them, so I left a message and went home to start the long holiday weekend. By the day after Thanksgiving, I was feeling unsettled about the delay if we ultimately decided to treat these two men, so I called the CDC again and asked the operator to put me in touch with the rabies-control officer on call.

After a few minutes, he answered and identified himself. I had met this man during my two-week training in Atlanta several months before, so I reintroduced myself, then told him I needed his advice about whether a particular circumstance involving human exposure to a now-proven rabid bat warranted treatment. He asked for the particulars, which I then recited to him. As I finished, I noted that if the bat had bitten the humans, the need for vaccine would be clear. But as it was the other way around, I needed him to help me decide whether a human biting a dead rabid bat constituted rabies exposure.

As I finished, there was a noticeable pause. Then he told me he'd actually met Dr. Jarvis, the state health officer in Nevada and had Dr. Jarvis's home telephone number in Reno. Further, he said he was about to hang up and immediately dial Dr. Jarvis's number in Reno and ask him about this alleged episode of man biting rabid bat.

And the line went dead.

I hung up the phone and waited. The phone rang a few seconds later, and I picked it up. A voice asked if I was Dr. Jarvis, state health officer of Nevada. After I indicated that I was indeed Dr. Jarvis, the CDC officer asked if I knew anything about a rabid bat being bitten by two men. Upon my response that, yes, I not only knew the story but had just told it to him, he audibly sighed.

He'd hoped he wouldn't actually need to answer the question, which was why he'd decided to check to see if this had been a crank call.

He apologized for interrupting the initial call and then began to ask more questions about the incident. Ultimately he begged me for some additional time to ask around among his fellow rabies control officers about how to respond to this inquiry. The advice that eventually was forthcoming was that little, if any, rabies exposure was likely to have occurred, but given the unusual circumstance, the rabies vaccine series should be offered.

This was no small recommendation for the Nevada Division of Health. Rabies vaccine doses were scarce in the state, principally because they cost so much. There was no budget set aside to cover these costs. I had enough doses already on hand in state control to begin the course of immunization for these two men but would need additional doses shipped to the state to finish. This was expensive—at least several thousand dollars. I was probably going to be constrained to bill these costs to the two men but was equally likely to receive absolutely no payment from them.

Nonetheless, I tried to get the men back on the telephone in order to explain my recommendation based on the advice from the CDC.

To my surprise, neither of the them wished to have the vaccine. They chose to risk developing the uniformly fatal consequence of rabies exposure, if that had occurred. So I didn't order any additional doses of the vaccine and finished the holiday weekend with at least a few undisturbed hours of family time.

When I arrived at my Carson City office the following Monday morning, I had multiple telephone messages from Austin. The first was from a woman whose name I didn't recognize. I placed a return call and discovered she was the common-law wife of one of the two men. She was frantically asking me if she could have the rabies injections. I asked her if she had participated in the night of revelry with the bat. None of the eyewitnesses with whom I'd spoken reported seeing any women along for the party, and she confirmed she had been nowhere near the bat.

In fact, she'd never seen the dead animal and had known nothing about the incident until the end of the Thanksgiving weekend. At that time, she'd been informed she was not going to be allowed to work at her job as a waitress unless and until she received the rabies immunizations, by order of the county attorney. Another of the messages was from the other common-law wife, who likewise had been ordered away from her job as a laundress until she completed the vaccinations.

Thus, a preposterous situation developed. Two men who'd had a pathetic, alcohol-fueled exposure to a dead rabid bat, each of them with a marginal risk for rabies, turned down the rabies vaccine despite a public-health recommendation to undergo immunization. But two women, neither of whom had ever seen the bat, but both of whom had had household and presumably sexual contact with the two men, had been placed on some kind of job quarantine by the local county attorney out of concern for rabies transmission. Another surreal Nevada moment. The purple world gone crazy.

Another telephone message on my desk that Monday morning was from the county attorney herself. She began the conversation grateful to me for bringing the rabies problem out into the open so she could act to protect the public. I responded that I was unaware how I'd brought the case into public purview since I'd never spoken with the press, or with her office, or any other elected official about the particulars of the case. She indicated that my having investigated the case by interviewing various eyewitnesses had been enough, since the local gossip was sufficient to carry the essential aspects of the matter to her ears.

Further, she knew that the two men had refused the necessary care and, in her opinion, had thereby placed the entire community at risk since they lived with women who had jobs that could expose the entire community. I asked her what she meant by that statement. She responded that, of course, these women could contract the disease from their common-law husbands and then pass the disease on through the food and laundry they might be contaminating.

At this point in the conversation, I determined to enlighten her and relieve her concern and allow everyone in Austin to move on. I pointed out that rabies was not a disease spread person to person through sexual contact, household contact, food-borne transmission, or contaminated clothing, doorknobs, or any other object. To emphasize this point, I told her that US cases were rare and only occurred when a human had direct contact with the saliva of an animal suffering from rabies, usually through a bite strong enough to break the skin.

To my surprise, none of this seemed of interest to the county attorney. She was convinced she was standing on a rampart defending her community from contagion, and nothing I said was going to alter her course. The women were not allowed to work until they finished a course of the rabies vaccine, period. She was quite unhappy with me for failing to support her cause.

I asked her if her office was prepared to pay for the vaccine. She was more than surprised that I would try to saddle her with the cost, particularly after she found out how much that cost would be. Her expectation was that my office would supply the vaccine; she didn't care to know how it was to be paid for. Unfortunately, I had no legal mechanism at my disposal to reverse her foolish quarantine, at least according to the Nevada deputy attorney general, to whom I placed my next phone call.

So I called the two women back, one at a time, and explained the situation to them. By this time, they couldn't be consoled, no matter how I tried to assure them they were at no risk for rabies. Not only were they frightened by rabies, they were scared they'd be ostracized and never be able to work in Austin again. They needed their jobs in order to make a living. Repeatedly, they pleaded for the vaccine. It was, from their point of view, their only option. So I ordered more doses to be shipped by express and arranged for the few doses I had on hand to be sent to the local public-health nurses to be dispensed to these two women. I warned them that they would be billed for the vaccine and the nursing time necessary for the injections, but I knew the health division would never be paid.

Two weeks later, with the women progressing through their various doses, both of the men suddenly became petrified that they too might get rabies. They called to insist they also receive vaccine. How could I refuse? So I ordered more vaccine and went to see the Nevada Division of Health financial officer to try to figure out how we might scrape together the necessary funds. He told me the total amount now paid out would require a visit with the interim Ways and Means Committee of the Nevada legislature.

We were spending money that had not been appropriated, and we would have to account for the expenditure. The committee met monthly, as I recall, and the health division was already on the agenda for spending beyond appropriations because we'd found a case of antibiotic-resistant tuberculosis that had required specialized care available only in Denver at the National Jewish Hospital, where the inpatient billed charges were enormous. That one case of TB cost several times more than the usual annual Nevada budget for tuberculosis control.

Paying for the real purple world in the United States is expensive enough. Care for cases such as antibiotic-resistant tuberculosis is beyond the fiscal capacity of almost every American household. Therefore, it's nonsense to suggest that we all, as individuals, need to come to terms with being financially responsible for our own health care. An appendectomy can cost upward of $15,000. How many American families can afford that? And yet, as a society, we can afford to make sure no one needs to die because they had appendicitis or antibiotic resistant TB. We should stop referring to efforts to pay for health care on a community-wide basis as socialism. No one can afford to build the roads they need either, so we join together as a community and construct highways, and we don't call them socialist superhighways.

There is no constitutional right to asphalt from my house to the White House, but we build highways anyway. Why? Because it's pragmatic and effective. The forty-seven thousand or so miles of interstate freeways in the United States were built at an original cost of just over $400 billion, just more than one-tenth of the annual cost of health care in the United States. Likewise, health care is pragmatic and needs an effective infrastructure for the American way of life in the twenty-first century. And let's not kid ourselves about Americans being able to make good choices through health-care shopping. American patients are as clueless about purchasing health care as the two drunk miners were about handling a dead bat.

Don't kid yourself either about whether one or the other of our major American political parties is more responsible for spouting nonsense about health care, like that county attorney fighting rabies transmission by protecting the community laundry. Let us be clear—both parties routinely violate what should be our nation's cherished values for health-care delivery: publicly paid health infrastructure enabling our pursuit of life, liberty, and happiness. Both political parties also routinely ignore the facts about American health-care delivery—that it's vastly more expensive than anywhere else on the planet precisely because it's the worst health-care system for patients in the first world. Red and blue politicians alike sanctimoniously shout at each other about health policy as if claiming pure motives for themselves and decrying the health policy of the opposing side. Meanwhile, they offer nearly identical visions of our health-care system (Romneycare, Obamacare, and now Trumpcare), which always serve the profit motives of the medical industrial complex. If you allow yourself to take sides in this partisan bickering, you're part of the problem.

Chapter Seven

Why Politicians Cannot Be Trusted

OST OF THE Nevada officials, elected and appointed, with whom I interacted, were uninformed about public-health science and didn't care to learn. They made policy based upon political calculations, like the county attorney in Austin who was hailed in her tiny town as a heroine because she (in their view) took a courageous stand against a pathetic state bureaucrat (that would be me). Never mind that her policy position was bereft of any science. She fed on the ignorance of her community.

Likewise, the director of prisons took what he viewed as a courageous stand, but one devoid of science. He had the political problem of appeasing the prison guards during a time when awareness of AIDS and HIV infection was generally increasing. Because of the prevalence of drug abuse among the inmates of the state penitentiary, the guards were persuaded that many of the men they encountered in their work at the penitentiary would be HIV positive.

Evidently, there was a growing fear among the guards that their occupation placed them at high risk for acquiring HIV infection. In one instance, I was called to the maximum-security facility in Carson City to examine a doorjamb that had allegedly been contaminated with human blood. Because the doorjamb was wooden, there was a concern that a splinter might jab a passing guard and infect him with HIV.

When the first request for this service came to me by telephone, I informed the caller, who was from the director's office, that there was no need for me to spend my time actually going to the prison. I stated that I knew without viewing the door that transmission of HIV would not occur through exposure to splinters. If there was concern about blood contaminating the door, I suggested the prison staff use a bleach solution to wipe it clean.

But the request was not withdrawn despite my definitive statement. The director of corrections simply arranged for a meeting in the governor's office. I was invited to the meeting to discuss the doorjamb with the director of prisons, the governor's chief of staff, with other dignitaries, and with Larry Matheis. The meeting was not convened solely to discuss door splinters in the prison system but rather the underlying concern about HIV transmission from inmates to guards.

The corrections department had decided the best policy would be to test each inmate for HIV as they entered the prison system and then test them again as they were paroled or otherwise released into the community. In the context of the discussion about this very expensive proposal, I was asked to tour the entire prison facility in order to get a proper perspective of the problems encountered at work by prison guards.

Though I objected to the proposed HIV surveillance of prisoners, I agreed to tour the prison. Of course, while I was there, the door in question was pointed out, and I was again asked about the risk it might represent for HIV transmission.

I opposed the prison HIV surveillance proposal principally because it would not protect the prison guards from whatever HIV exposure, if any, would occur at their workplace. The prison needed to implement universal blood and bodily fluid protections, not test inmates. But I also believed that the real intent was to allow prison guards to know which of the prisoners might happen to be HIV positive so that the guards could handle those persons differently. I doubted the HIV positive prisoners would get help with their infection. And I doubted the information would be kept confidential. Further, since the proposal included HIV testing during both admission to prison and release, it occurred to me that the surveillance program would identify people who acquired HIV infection while in the custody of the state of Nevada, thereby potentially revealing the failure of the state prison system to keep inmates from practicing the behaviors associated with HIV transmission, specifically IV drug use and penetrating sexual activity.

In making objections to the proposal, I failed to perceive the role I was expected to play. No one was asking me for my opinion about testing state prison inmates for HIV. That decision had already been made. Nothing short of my complete endorsement was anticipated because I was supposed to care more about the health of the prison guards and less about the health of the inmates. Public health and medicine cannot make that distinction while maintaining a place on moral high ground. Everybody's health matters. On principle, the health of each person matters more than the profitability of the medical industrial complex.

I'd obviously failed to make that point to the director of prisons. However, the prison system implemented the surveillance program, nonetheless. I don't know if or how HIV-positive prisoners might have suffered once they were discovered through this surveillance program. I know that they didn't receive HIV-related medical treatment, at least while I was employed by Nevada.

A year or so later, I was able to get the prison medical department to allow my designee to review the HIV-surveillance data dealing with the prison inmates. I asked an officer from the CDC to come to Nevada and conduct the review. By the time the review took place, over one thousand inmates had received HIV testing as they entered prison and as they were released, with only two individuals converting from a negative HIV test at first to a positive test upon exit.[7] Thus, in some ways, perhaps the gamble taken by the Nevada Corrections Department paid off, assuming they were able to assuage the fears of their guards while demonstrating that HIV seroconversion in prison was a rare event.

Too often, health-care interventions in the United States serve a purpose remote from the health of people. Sometimes it is to satisfy unfounded fears. Most often, that purpose is to make a profit.

In a related episode, the state professional association for firefighters and emergency responders felt that they were at risk for HIV infection when providing mouth-to-mouth resuscitation. So they hired a lobbyist to assist them with legislation requiring their employers to provide them with disposable pocket masks to be used over the mouths of people requiring CPR.

The lobbyist didn't even consider inquiring with the Nevada Division of Health about the need for this extra cost or whether the use of face masks would really reduce risk for HIV among EMS personnel. The first I heard of the bill during the 1989 legislative session was when a hearing for it was "noticed up" on the assembly side. I discussed the bill with Myla Florence, who by then was the division administrator, and she gave me permission to attend the hearing and speak. As per custom, I registered with the clerk of the committee upon arrival and indicated my intent to provide testimony.

The lobbyist, anticipating I would be helpful to her cause, introduced herself. She was manifestly unhappy with me when I told her that I considered this proposal to be a useless gesture in the prevention of the spread of HIV and therefore not a justifiable expense, small as it may be. But she needn't have worried. The assembly committee couldn't have been less interested in what the Nevada state health officer had to say about the matter. The legislation passed easily, and the lobbyist bragged about besting me at the legislative hearing.

But it's not to her credit, or anyone's for that matter, when fear replaces real values and facts in the setting of health policy. Labels applied to health policy, untrue though they may be, like "death panels" and "socialism," seem to uniformly inject fear and loathing into what should be reasoned discussion about what we as Americans value and know about health care we so generously fund for ourselves and our children. These fears then distract us from the real problems of our health-care system. We're so distracted, in fact, that most Americans can't begin to recite the basic principles and facts about how and why we seek good care.

Fortunately, that bill was not the only AIDS-related legislation passed in 1989. The state AIDS Task Force had, with the prodding of Larry Matheis, written substantive legislation about communicable disease control for consideration during the session. The task force co-chairs had become, respectively, the senate and assembly sponsors of this bill. It was, in essence, a massive rewrite of the statutes concerning public-health authority to make Nevada a little less purple. Assemblyman Sedway, who was not a member of the AIDS Task Force, took a personal interest in the bill and helped it along.

He was all for an attempt to induce some order in the public-health statutes when it came to communicable disease control. I became more involved with the task force after Larry Matheis left the health division in late 1988 to become executive director of the Nevada State Medical Association, where he has served effectively ever since.

In 1989, I took on the task of summarizing the AIDS epidemic in Nevada after Larry had been responsible for publishing the data in 1987 and 1988. Ultimately I was invited to submit an article about AIDS and HIV in Nevada to the *Western Journal of Medicine*.[8] By then, Governor Bryan had left for Washington, DC, and Lt. Governor Bob Miller had been sworn in as his replacement.

The Miller administration was strict in its requirement that state employees were not to offer requests for appropriations not approved through the governor's budget. Despite that warning—and noting that Nevada had the seventh highest incidence of AIDS in the nation but as yet no state appropriation for the prevention and treatment of HIV related disease—I asked Mr. Sedway during a private conversation to look for funds to place in the AIDS treatment budget. The AIDS treatment budget was newly created by the legislation sponsored by the AIDS task force.

I think he tried, but Nevada ended up with an AIDS budget category without any funding, at least in 1989. I didn't remain in office long enough to find out whether the new communicable disease statute actually gave the state health officer a stronger hand in making the state of Nevada less purple. As a nation, our real values are shown in our government budgets. What we spend tax money on is what we really care about. By that measure, we really do care about health services. Unfortunately, we're allowing both red and blue politicians to steal these generous funds for profiteering (another purple world).

Medicare Advantage plans are private-sector health-insurance benefits for senior citizens funded at a higher cost with tax money intended for the Medicare program. Medicare Part D, the mechanism for purchasing medications for senior Americans eligible for Medicare, cannot, by law, negotiate best prices for drugs. For that reason, these drugs cost on average 60 percent more in the United States than they should. Durable medical equipment, like powered wheelchairs, can be seen on television advertising to Medicare enrollees to be guaranteed covered, no matter the cost. On a bipartisan basis, elected federal officials are willing to give the medical industrial complex whatever it wants from the generous tax funding of health-care services. This must stop.

Where Mr. Sedway had no sympathy with public-health efforts, however, was in tobacco control. He was a three-pack-a-day smoker despite the fact that he'd had two major heart attacks and survived the removal of one lung due to lung cancer. Politicians, remember, cannot be trusted, and sometimes that is because they are crazily inconsistent human beings.

During one of the Ways and Means Committee hearings in 1989, he set his beard on fire with his cigarette. The flames were extinguished by one of his committee colleagues who spotted the fire first and threw a cup of coffee on Mr. Sedway. During my first public-health investigation, I'd encountered Mr. Sedway's strong feelings about the freedom smokers should enjoy. Almost as soon as I arrived in Nevada, I received a complaint that the building housing the state legislature was "sick." I was instructed that I must respond, investigate, and make recommendations.

Having at that time recently come from OSHA, I was dimly aware of the then rapidly growing interest nationwide in "sick-building syndrome," which was the term then in use to describe nonspecific eye, nose, and throat irritation among the occupants of a problem building. The National Institute of Occupational Safety and Health (NIOSH), part of the Centers for Disease Control, had been conducting health-hazard evaluations in various office buildings around the nation in response to complaints just like the one I received about the legislature's home building.

Mostly, the investigators concluded that indoor tobacco smoke was irritating nonsmoking building occupants. Naturally, I thought I might be able to get a NIOSH investigation underway in Carson City. What I discovered, however, was that NIOSH had been inundated with requests for building investigations to the point the staff were simply unable to respond any further. Instead, staff at NIOSH provided me with a copy of their protocol for conducting these investigations, and I was on my own.

One of the initial steps in such an investigation was to meet with the significant decision makers in the building to outline the proposed investigation in order to elicit their cooperation.

The owners of the building were, in effect, the assembly and senate of Nevada, each housed in one half of the structure. During the fall of 1987, when I started the investigation, the legislature was not in session. Consequently, the building was only minimally occupied, very much unlike what had occurred during the session early in the year when the complaint had been generated.

There was, therefore, not much point in spending money on indoor environmental testing. But I did meet with some legislators who, because they were in leadership, were actually occasionally on site, including Mr. Sedway. When I walked into his office armed with the data from NIOSH about how secondhand tobacco smoke was a major cause of indoor air pollution, I found him chain smoking under a sign hung on his office wall that said, "If you disagree with my freedom to smoke, you are free to leave."

He was the principle reason why the assembly half of the legislative building had no policy restricting smoking. The Nevada Senate, on the other hand, strictly forbade smoking anywhere in the rooms they controlled. The line of delineation was strictly enforced, to the degree that any doors between the two halves of the building were kept locked. The air-handling systems for the two sides of the building were mostly, but not entirely, separated. Not surprisingly, therefore, the nonsmoking staff members on the senate side of the building reported (through questionnaires that I circulated) a greater degree of well-being while at their work stations than did the nonsmoking staff of the assembly.

Given that Mr. Sedway refused to consider a change in indoor smoking wherever he had control, my report concerning indoor air pollution at the Nevada State Legislative Building made very little difference.

I found that the offices of the Nevada State Health Division, including the public-health nursing clinics where pregnant women and infants received services, were all full of tobacco smoke. Indeed, everywhere in Nevada, as a matter of public policy, both private and public buildings were considered smoking areas unless alternative arrangements had been made.

It occurred to me that the statewide indoor air policy should be reversed: all public and private buildings should be considered nonsmoking unless alternative arrangements had been made. Larry Matheis agreed. He and I found the process to designate state health division offices statewide as nonsmoking to be arduous, though he eventually succeeded.

I think Larry arranged for me to speak to an interim health committee of the legislature about indoor air quality and tobacco smoke. I prepared and gave a review of the US surgeon general's report on the subject, augmented by a then-recent publication from the Environmental Protection Agency. It is now well-accepted science that tobacco smoke is far more dangerous than the purple world of microbiological disease.

My presentation generated no small amount of discussion, principally because the lobbyist representing Big Tobacco asked for and was granted time to respond to my presentation. He framed the issue, of course, in terms of personal freedom, ignoring the fact that a nonsmoker was not free to not smoke when sitting near someone who smoked. And he played to the gaming industry, citing what was always said about gamblers: that they liked to smoke and would not come to a casino where the use of tobacco was regulated or prohibited. This was a self-fulfilling prophecy, in my opinion. In fact, I remember seeing some tourism survey information that indicated that a majority of first-time gaming tourists from out of state were nonsmokers who indicated that the smoke in the casinos was a deterrent to repeat visits.

In other words, if the gaming experience were to become friendlier to nonsmokers, then more nonsmokers would frequent the casinos. The irony of this presentation from the tobacco lobbyist was that he was already at that time dying of cancer, probably smoking induced. Marvin Sedway also died of smoking-induced cancer. He developed cancer in his remaining lung and, of course, could have no surgical cure.

Lung cancer was, at that time, becoming increasingly common in Las Vegas. Nevada's population had close to the highest rate of smoking in the nation. We knew this because one of the programs from the Centers for Disease Control I did manage to start for the first time in Nevada was the Behavioral Risk Factor Surveillance Survey (BRFSS).

All forty-nine other states had already been multiyear participants in this random telephone survey of their citizens sponsored and paid for by the CDC. They provided not only funds but also technical expertise to support this gathering of information about the personal habits of each state's citizens that could be risk factors for chronic diseases, such as cancer, heart attack, stroke, diabetes, and emphysema, or injuries.

The CDC created the questionnaire, helped train the personnel who would administer the questionnaire by random-digit telephone dialing, and processed the data for us. We merely wrote a grant for the funds needed to pay for the labor and other costs of actually calling Nevadans and asking them the questions.

I was allowed to add a question or two to the previously organized list of queries. I chose to ask each respondent whether he or she had health insurance or some other mechanism for financing needed health care and discovered that one in five Nevadans had no health-care financing at all (a high percentage, though not the highest rate of uninsured among the fifty United States).

We also discovered that Nevadans are unlikely to wear seat belts and are very likely to be binge drinkers, smokers, and have unhealthy diets. Of course, most of the people living in Nevada were actually born and raised somewhere else. During the late 1980s, there were just over one million Nevadans, as I recall. But by then there had been less than one million births ever registered in Nevada throughout its history. Thus, the smoking habits and consequent risk for lung cancer for at least a plurality of residents, maybe even the majority, were established elsewhere and, as people migrated to the state, principally to Las Vegas, during adulthood.

The rising rate of lung cancer was not, strictly speaking, a native Nevada issue, particularly given the fact that lung cancer takes decades to develop from the onset of smoking to the manifestation of symptoms.

This fact, however, didn't stop people in Nevada from pointing the finger for cancers of all types at their favorite environmental hazard, whatever that may have been in their individual part of the state. In Southern Nevada, most of the environmental faultfinding was laid on the federal government because of the presence of the Nevada Test Site, located less than one hundred miles north of Las Vegas. People in Nevada and Utah have, for many years now, commonly called themselves "downwinders," referring to being downwind of the open-air nuclear-bomb testing that occurred at the Nevada Test Site until a few years before I served as the state health officer.

I was invited to observe an underground nuclear explosion at the site while still in the employ of the state health division. The explosion was set to go off very early one morning. The day before the scheduled event, Myla Florence and I were invited to tour the entire Nevada Test Site.

We were taken five miles underground to look at the preparations underway for a future "shot," as the test explosions were commonly called. A great deal of time and effort went into observing that milliseconds' worth of a nuclear explosion before the inferno melted all the machinery. The fireball would then raise the desert floor above and melt the rock below, eventually leaving a visible depression.

I saw some aboveground film footage of previous "shoots" that left the impression that small jets of dust escaped the blast into the atmosphere. Perhaps because of that small potential for gas or dust release, the weather had to be just right before a shoot would actually go forward. No wind toward Las Vegas was permitted. The shoot I had come to witness was cancelled because of the direction of the prevailing winds.

But the most bizarre part of the tour was driving around the vast

Nevada Test Site to see the remnants of the aboveground tests. There were a series of holes in the ground due to experiments that used nuclear bombs as an excavation technique. Adjustments were made in the size of the bomb and the height off the ground of the explosion in order to optimize the size of the hole.

The largest hole was a half mile deep and a mile wide. I am completely unclear about what purpose such an excavation might serve; it seemed too big for a basement. Additionally, we were not allowed to approach the hole because it remained too radioactive, then more than twenty years after the "dig."

Then there was a series of fake towns complete with buildings, streets, bridges, and other structures all in various contorted, melted, and obliterated conditions. Apparently the point of that series of explosions was to determine the effects of nuclear explosions on modern infrastructure. It seemed to me that question had been answered in Japan in 1945.

The apparent silliness of the open-air testing programs, however, does not amount to saying that exposure to radioactivity from the atmospheric testing was the cause of cancer in those living downwind.

Dr. Daniel W. Miles, himself a downwinder, has published exhaustive reviews of the science concerning both exposure to radioactivity and cancer rates among the alleged downwind populations. He is careful in the way he words his final assessment: "People find the discussion of fallout-induced cancer deaths almost irreverent. The author [Miles] can sympathize with this point of view. The discussion is not pleasant. On the other hand, we are facing situations where we need to know precisely the risks involved in radiation exposure. . . . The author has lingering doubts about whether fallout caused (cancer deaths)."[9]

Making a fuss about cancer among downwinders is much like deciding that rabies is a sexually transmitted disease. The world is purple enough from real threats to health. We should not be ignoring facts just because we fear what color our lives may be.

When it comes to health policy, most Americans are as confusing as

Marvin Sedway. He very much wanted to contribute to bringing Nevada into the (then) twentieth century in public health and in many other ways. However, he had a major personal failing: he couldn't give up smoking, even though that habit had caused him heart attacks, cancer, and he'd nearly burned himself. His inability to quit killed him, of course, but not before he negatively impacted many other's lives. He made the legislative staff members on the assembly side of the legislative building suffer with sick-building syndrome. He hampered efforts to make public-health clinics and offices smoke free. He valued his freedom to smoke more than the greater good of freeing Nevadans from the harm of inhaling carcinogens.

We Americans have similarly screwed up our nation with an irrational mix of health-care fears and falsehoods. We keep trying out crazy health-system experiments, like managed competition, accountable care organizations, and the donut hole in Medicare Part D. These Rube Goldberg policies are like attempting to excavate with nuclear bombs. We end up leaving behind an eerie, fake health-system skyline as witness to our folly. We are only burning and bombing ourselves.

Let's no longer fear that which cannot really hurt us. We pay for health care principally with taxes because we Americans value what health care can do for us. Our individual health is the necessary prerequisite for our pursuit of life, liberty, and happiness—the quintessential American dream. Let us fear the health-system pilfering, profiteering, and killing American patients while costing us our future fiscal health.

Chapter Eight

The Medical Industrial Complex:
It's All about the High-Priced Sale, Not the Patient

N NEVADA, THE hysteria regarding radiation exposure completely turned the state's initial interest in becoming the host for high-level nuclear waste storage. By the time I moved to Nevada, Yucca Mountain, a ridge just west of the Nevada Test Site, had been identified as one of three possible places in the United States for high-level radioactive waste storage, needed as a permanent repository for spent nuclear fuel rods.

In the 1987 Nevada legislative session, a new county was created that included the Yucca Mountain area. Property tax rates for the new county, called Bullfrog County, were intentionally set high by the legislature as a method for collecting as much money as possible from the federal project, which was then anticipated at Yucca Mountain.

The federal legislation creating the nuclear-waste repository included a provision for Payment Equal to Taxes (PETT) funding for the county that was the home of the nuclear repository. The PETT funding, as it was originally crafted by Congress, would bypass the state government, which rankled Nevada officials. So they created a new county, but one that had no people living in it, and declared in the legislation passed at the very last second of the 1987 Nevada legislative session that the county seat was many miles away in Carson City, the capital of Nevada.

All PETT funding (potentially as much as $25 million per year) for the new county would therefore go directly to the state government. Then governor Richard Bryan, the governor at the time I began my public-health service in Nevada, signed the bill into law.

Of course, later, during his 1988 run for the US Senate, he campaigned on a platform of refusing to allow the US government to build the repository in Nevada. He'd realized how easy it was to get votes when opposing anything nuclear. Utah's politicians have been using this same formula against the low-level nuclear waste site west of Salt Lake City for years. This begs the question that if politicians can use fear of ionizing radiation and its effect on health to get elected, even when invoked unscientifically, why can't we elect politicians who invoke fear of the health issues caused by legitimate problems in our health-care system?

Perhaps more importantly for Governor Bryan, an unpopulated county turned out to be unconstitutional, and so the 1989 Nevada legislature had to abolish Bullfrog County. Nevadans have strongly opposed the Yucca Mountain waste site ever since, even though not a single case of cancer in the state can legitimately be ascribed to any environmental radioactive contamination.

Not that there weren't any environmental disasters in Nevada. In the late 1980s, the Carson River was plagued by contamination. Birds and fish harvested from the river contained potentially harmful quantities of mercury. The environmental agency in the Nevada state government asked me to issue a warning about the consumption of game caught anywhere near the Carson River, which they thought would be taken more seriously if it came from the state health officer. If I remember correctly, I crafted wording that targeted pregnant women and children, warning them that developing nervous systems could be harmed by mercury exposure, which could be the consequence of eating game fish and birds from the Carson River Valley. The mercury had leached into the river over the many decades since the mining of silver in and around Virginia City, uphill from the Carson River.

But mining was not the only human activity that was hazardous to the Carson River system. Alfalfa farming was a big business around the downstream end of the river, which flows from the Sierra Nevada into the Great Basin and ends in vast wetlands. The alfalfa was grown to provide hay for California race horses, or so I was told back then. Of course, there is not enough rainfall to water alfalfa in Northern Nevada, so the crops were irrigated with water that flowed out of and then back into the Carson River. In the process, these waters became substantially more saline.

By the time I was working in Nevada, the rising salinity in combination with drought conditions was ruining the wetlands. I was invited to take an aerial tour of the Stillwater National Wildlife Refuge, one of the most important birding areas in North America supporting the millions of animals that migrate north and south each year. At the time of my tour, 90 percent of the seventy thousand or so acres of the refuge had turned brown, with millions of fish killed as the wetlands dried up and the remaining waters became too salty to support life, either animal or vegetable.

Fortunately, I believe there has been some reprieve for this international wildlife treasure as government agencies have purchased water rights from farmers and returned the flow of pristine streams back into the wetlands, reviving them. Please note that this example proves that government agencies can in fact turn major problems around and protect important resources.

The most significant environmental damage I remember seeing in Nevada in the late 1980s, however, was the damage associated with gold mining. Only low-grade gold ore was to be found in the Silver State, but with gold prices sustainably high, mining and refining the ore became very profitable. During the summer, various large mining interests would scavenge the high desert in the Great Basin looking for possible ore. Thousands of bags of rocks were sent to mineral laboratories to be assayed for precious-metal content. The rocks were ground to a fine powder, and the samples were geographically mapped so that the best sites could be exploited for ore. Dust exposure in the mineral assay laboratories was high.

I know this because two cases of congestive heart failure in young men were reported to me by the heart-transplant service in Salt Lake City prior to my resignation as state health officer. The two men worked for two different mineral assay laboratories in the Reno area. At my request, both laboratories were visited by an industrial hygienist employed by the Nevada Division of Occupational Health (Nevada's OSHA).

He reported high levels of dust from the rock-crushing operation at both facilities. Both men had rapid-onset heart failure caused by a non-inflammatory cardiomyopathy, which was likely caused not by the purple world of infection but by some kind of toxic exposure. One of the two men was so seriously ill he underwent heart transplantation in Salt Lake City. His surgeon, noting that two cases had suddenly appeared from Reno with a similar life-threatening illness, called to ask whether they could have been exposed to something toxic at work.

A computer-based literature review revealed that heavy metals can damage the heart muscle. During the 1960s in the United States, there was a particularly interesting series of congestive heart failure cases associated with cobalt exposure. Initially, the problem was called beer-drinkers' cardiomyopathy because heavy imbibers of brew began to experience the problem during that decade. But it was soon realized that only those beer drinkers who ingested brew laced with cobalt were actually at risk.

Cobalt had been added to some beer recipes once it was discovered that the metal stabilized the foam at the top of a glass of beer. Not being a beer drinker myself, I have no idea why that should be such an important property. But because it was, enough cobalt-laced beer was sold in the United States that an outbreak of what came to be known as cobalt cardiomyopathy was documented. Once the cardiotoxicity of cobalt was studied and understood, some researchers even began using cobalt as a method to induce heart failure in laboratory animals so that various remedies for heart failure could be studied, putting this discovery to good use.

Knowing that cobalt and perhaps some other metals could cause heart muscle damage (cardiomyopathy), and knowing that ores containing gold could also contain other metals, such as cobalt, and further, knowing that these two men had worked in assay laboratories where they had been heavily exposed to rocks that had been crushed to a fine powder and which probably contained metals, I hypothesized that these two cases of heart failure could be due to toxic workplace exposure.

The heart transplant team in Salt Lake City had heart tissue from both men, as well as heart tissue from other residents of Reno who had non-inflammatory cardiomyopathy but had not worked in the mineral assay industry. With help from former colleagues at federal OSHA, I found a laboratory able to measure metal content in heart tissue, and we compared the values in these various Reno heart cases.

Cobalt levels were extraordinarily high in the two heart-tissue samples from these two subject cases but not high in the comparison cases. This study was published in the *Journal of Occupational Medicine*.[10] This was one outbreak investigation I conducted without the assistance of the Centers for Disease Control.

Gold mining in Nevada is a big business, with over $228 billion (2011 prices) in gold extracted through 2008. But it didn't really take off on a massive scale until gold prices jumped substantially in the 1970s. The reason is simple: gold ore in Nevada is very low-grade, perhaps one part gold per million parts waste rock.

Therefore, a successful gold-mining operation in Nevada must move millions of tons of rock in order to realize a relatively small amount of gold. What makes this industry more profitable is that gold miners, unlike coal and oil extractors, do not pay royalties for extracting this precious metal from public lands in the United States because they are protected from this obligation by the General Mining Act of 1872. Additionally, in Nevada, the mining industry doesn't generally need to respond to anyone concerned about the environmental effects of their open-pit mining or cyanide leaching because elected officials in Nevada did not consider adverse environmental impacts a factor to weigh against the economic growth generated by mining.

While serving as the public-health leader in Nevada, I was invited to tour the gold mine and refining facilities located at Jerritt Canyon, north of Elko. Since the late 1980s, when I took the tour, this mine has changed hands and is now extracting ore underground. Some of the changes made to the mine, I believe, were induced because of litigation against the mine owner brought by the state of Idaho, which is downstream. What I saw in the 1980s was a massive dirt-moving operation, with trucks rolling on tires many feet in diameter, higher than I am tall.

The canyon was virtually filled in with the waste rock and soil from what had once been a neighboring mountain. After the ore had been crushed, it was laid out on vast leaching fields, acres wide, where it would be sprinkled with a cyanide solution that would dissolve the gold from the ore. The so-called "pregnant" cyanide solution was then collected so that the gold could be harvested. The leftover solution was collected in large ponds where waterfowl would mistakenly land and die.

This and other similar mining operations in Northern Nevada were sparking the economy of Elko and other small towns. Housing was at a premium, jobs were plentiful, and public projects were being funded and experiencing growth. The economic activity accounted for the paucity of repercussions against the environmental damage done. When dollars are to be made in Nevada, damages to people or the environment are not counted; they are expected and embraced. Another kind of purple world similar to that of extracting handsome profits in health care by mining the illnesses and injuries suffered by Americans.

Indeed, the caricature of American free enterprise that has always been business as usual in Nevada has taken over American health-care delivery. Just because gambling, prostitution, and raping the landscape to extract precious metals can be profitable does not make these activities good. In fact, what is profitable, if it comes at the expense of what is humane or divine, actually devalues rather than enriches us. Just so in American health-care delivery. We would rather sell more drugs or surgeries than actually care for people. American shoppers are quite savvy when it comes to hunting bargains in the marketplace of commodities, from cars to cantaloupes. But the buyer of health care is not a shopper; he or she is a patient. By definition, a patient is not positioned to take time to consider options before making a purchase. It's the twisted logic of American health policy that American patients should have "skin in the game" when it comes to health-care purchases.

One other episode I experienced as the state health officer involving Nevada's dirt deserves mention. As the state health officer, I automatically became the food and drug commissioner for the state as well. Mostly, this additional title meant I could condemn improperly handled food, such as when a refrigerated trailer was damaged while crossing the desert and the truck driver tried to salvage something of his investment by selling the now-thawing meat on the side of the highway (yes, this actually happened).

But, as indicated in that title, I was also the regulatory authority for "drugs" made and sold in Nevada. Pharmaceutical firms generally make their products for sale across state lines and are therefore subject to federal regulation due to the "Interstate Commerce Clause" of the US Constitution. But within an individual state, laws can be passed that regulate the manufacture and sale of "drugs" without federal oversight.

Two such drugs—Laetrile and Gerovatal—had received special legislative approval in Nevada. Laetrile was supposed to have remarkable anticancer properties. These properties never seemed to be manifest when this chemical, a derivative of apricot pits, was subjected to real clinical testing.

But the Nevada legislature is not particularly concerned about clinical science and thus approved the manufacture and sale of Laetrile, subject to the regulation of the food and drug commissioner (without giving said commissioner any staffing or funding for actually doing anything, as usual). Gerovatal was a simple chemical compound with local anesthetic properties that was said to reverse the aging process.

The legislative sponsor of the bill making it legal to manufacture and sell Gerovatal in Nevada stated in his testimony in support of the legislation that after taking this remarkable pill, he'd been able to drive the golf ball fifty yards farther off the tee.

Sounds persuasive to me.

I took very little interest in the manufacture and sale of these two non-FDA approved "medications." However, at one point I was assailed by someone claiming to be the sole "real" manufacturer of Gerovatal. He was upset because I was not properly regulating the manufacture of this substance. He claimed that another company was making false Gerovatal and selling it to an unsuspecting public. My initial response was to tell him that there was no way for anyone to know which Gerovatal was true and which was false, since neither could reverse human aging anyway.

He was not pleased with, nor did he find any humor in, that remark. So, by way of looking into this problem, I sent an inspector to a retail outlet selling the various brands of Gerovatal and had him purchase the two different kinds. These were then tested by a state facility. The "true" product indeed contained the so-called active chemical ingredient. The "false" product was just a capsule full of good-old Nevada desert dirt. This discovery led to a request that the offending manufacturer simply be shut down. This, of course, would have been a potentially difficult thing to do and certainly would have required that the state attorney assigned to the division of health be prepared to litigate.

He felt the litigation would be time- and resource consuming without any real impact on public health and welfare. So instead I simply told the manufacturer of the "false" Gerovatal that he could not call his product by that name. He complied, changing the name of his product to Geravatal. The "true" manufacturer of Gerovatal was not at all satisfied by this outcome, but I simply said that if Nevada customers were so foolish as to believe that either brand (Gerovatal or Geravatal) could actually reverse aging, they'd be as well served by consuming a capsule of Nevada dirt as they would a capsule of local anesthetic.

Case closed.

These are not just quaint anecdotes about pharmacological nonsense in Nevada. The manufacture and sale of medications in America is big business and increasingly has little to do with improving patient health. Americans are assailed by commercial speech touting the advantages of various drugs all the time, always with a rapid staccato disclaimer at the end of the ad, as if anyone could possibly absorb the information. Patients need new antibiotics, but none are being developed. Why? Because a good antibiotic is generally taken over no more than a two-week course, which could never be the basis of a blockbuster marketing breakthrough for Big Pharma.

We don't need more copycat drugs, for instance, to treat heartburn. But we get them, like one called the Purple Pill, because heartburn is common, and once someone starts taking such a drug they will likely take it for many months, even years. Cancer is perhaps the most feared disease in America, though it is not one disease but many. Cancer chemotherapy seems to offer hope in one of life's most difficult moments. What patient can actually make a reasoned decision about which, if any, cancer agent to swallow? These decisions are never made by the patient, which explains why prices for the newer chemotherapies are ranging well into the thousands of dollars *per dose*.

Fear of cancer drives demand for even the slightest hope in treatment, no matter what the price. In health care, unlike in a real market, there is no inverse relationship between price and demand. FDA approval requires that drug companies demonstrate both the safety and efficacy of new treatments. Why? Because patients don't know the difference between a safe and effective treatment and snake oil. We need a strong public-health presence protecting our patients from pharmaceutical fraud. And we need a payer for health services strong enough to push back when, as happened recently, the price for a drug increases overnight by 5,000 percent. This kind of business as usual, profit-taking approach to health-care delivery is killing patients in the United States. Surely the vast majority of Americans can agree that human life is more valued and important than a corporate business plan.

Chapter Nine

American Health Care:
High Profit, Poor Quality

THERE ARE MANY categories of health and disease for which statistics are kept in the United States, including communicable diseases (whether sexually transmitted, food or water borne, vector borne, or preventable by vaccine or whatever); chronic diseases (cancer, heart disease, chronic lung or liver damage); and injuries (whether intentional, self-inflicted, or road related).

In many of these categories, Nevadans bear a burden greater than the citizenry of almost all other states. Yet few in Nevada seem interested in investigating why this may be or what can be done to improve the health of the state's residents.

For instance, at the time I was state health officer, Nevada had the highest suicide rate in the United States. This was at a time when the CDC had recently organized a new branch with the purpose of studying the causes of injury in the United States, including risk factors related to suicide.

As the Nevada state health officer, my last request to the CDC for epidemiology assistance was to the injury-control branch. I asked them to send a team of investigators to study the high rate of suicide in Nevada. Soon after the CDC team arrived in Nevada, they were featured in a news conference by the then new governor, Bob Miller. He seemed genuinely interested in furthering the understanding of suicide as a public-health problem.

The CDC team set about a carefully planned agenda, gathering data about the frequency of suicide in Nevada and the frequency of suicide ideation and attempts among college freshmen at the University of Nevada in Reno. College freshmen were studied because it was easy to find them and they were of an age with the highest risk for suicide.

This study confirmed many previously hypothesized risk factors for suicide. For instance, suicide is more common among the aged and the adolescent, completed suicide is more common for males, and social isolation is often an antecedent to suicide. But different from the study of suicide elsewhere, in Nevada—among the significant findings of the investigation, as I recall—was an association between working for a casino and suicide. Gaming employment is a large share of the job market in Nevada.

This finding was clearly unwelcome.

By the time the results of the study were published, I'd already resigned from the Nevada Division of Health, though I was still living in Reno. I remember being interviewed by a Utah radio station about the results of the investigation, but not by any media outlet in Nevada. Governor Miller, who was given a copy of the report, never mentioned it, to my knowledge. And, not surprisingly, the Nevada Division of Health followed his lead.

Fortunately, it seems the state of Nevada has, at least in some regards, outgrown this lack of interest in public health. For instance, credit is due to public-health workers in subsequent Nevada administrations for their efforts to fund suicide prevention. There is now a Suicide Prevention Project within the Nevada state government. Progress has been made.

Shortly after the CDC suicide-investigation findings became available, I was hired by a Nevada law firm as an expert witness on issues related to suicide in Nevada. These lawyers were defending a recording company in a lawsuit filed by the families of two young men. The men in question had listened to some rock music that allegedly glorified suicide—and then they'd gone to a school yard and shot themselves, one dying, the other surviving with half his face blown off.

I was being asked to describe and explain the data I'd induced the CDC to create about the possible causes of Nevada's high rate of suicide.

This data was to cast doubt on the plaintiff's assertion that suicide is directly caused by listening to rock music, so it was relevant to the issues at trial.

Due to a pretrial settlement, I was never called to provide sworn testimony in the matter. Though providing expert testimony has, since then, become a significant part of my professional life.

In fact, the first experience I had with expert testimony occurred while I was serving as Nevada's chief health officer. I was asked by lawyers who worked for the US Department of Labor to serve as an expert witness in a New York City trial that concerned some OSHA violations.

Before leaving the US Department of Labor in Washington, DC, to accept the appointment in Nevada, I'd reviewed medical surveillance data acquired by OSHA inspectors at a mercury recycling plant in New York. At the plant, old thermometers were crushed so that the mercury could be captured and recycled. Unfortunately, proper control of mercury exposure had not been organized, and the employees at the plant had a history of mercury toxicity.

The plant was required to organize better exposure controls and to instigate medical surveillance for mercury poisoning symptoms and signs. As a medical officer for OSHA, I was asked to review the medical surveillance data and render an opinion about whether it indicated the employees might be overexposed to the metal. In fact, elevated urine mercury levels were documented in the data, as were the signs of poisoning, such as tremors.

Based in part on my opinion, the OSHA field officers had issued citations to the employer for violations of workplace safety standards, to which the employer had objected, thus creating the need for an administrative law trial, which was held in the World Trade Center.

After I was examined by the US attorney handling the case, the defense attorney wanted to get on record that I was being paid for my testimony. Through this, he hoped to reduce my credibility. What he didn't know was that Larry Matheis had agreed to give me time off from my Nevada work in order to respond to the federal request for my expert testimony in the case—with the proviso that I could not bill the US government for my professional services. Larry felt that a public-health official should not be receiving extra funds for performing a public service. He noted that I knew about the case because of my previous employment with the US Department of Labor. Since I had been a public servant then and continued to be so as the state health officer of Nevada, he expected that I would render testimony without extra remuneration.

So when the defense attorney cross-examined me under oath and asked me to tell the judge what my fee would be for appearing in court, he was quite surprised to discover I would not be billing for my time. He made a comment about how I must be the only altruistic doctor in the nation, or something to that effect. His comment probably reflects the growing opinion of Americans that doctors and other health professionals are into making serious money as their first professional objective. And I'm sad to say, there is some truth to this increasing cynicism.

Doctors do take gifts, small and large, from pharmaceutical agents in exchange for opportunities to place prescriptions. Some doctors invest in the very institutions and instruments they use in their practice, creating the real possibility that they make referrals or admissions based more on possible reimbursement than on doing what's best for patient care. To be fair, medical-education debt is often quite large and not something a brand-new physician can ignore. It took me twenty years to pay off the debts I incurred as a medical student.

Personally, I'm persuaded that altruism among medical and health professionals remains an effective motivation. One of the twentieth century's most illustrious surgeons, Dr. Edward Delos Churchill of Massachusetts General Hospital once said: "Charity in the broad spiritual sense—the desire to relieve suffering . . . is the most precious possession of medicine."[11] Those of us who've been blessed with the opportunity to know the gratitude of a patient can understand what Dr. Churchill was trying to say about the practice of medicine.

As mentioned previously, perhaps the most important discovery ever made and which ushered in the modern era of treating infectious disease (and made the world far less purple) was the chance observation by Sir Alexander Fleming that a chemical released from a *Penicillium* mold could kill certain disease-causing bacteria. It took nearly twenty years from the initial lab discovery before penicillin could be mass-produced and used, which it was for the first time as a treatment for wounded Allied soldiers on D-Day.

Fleming received the Nobel Prize for his observation, but he was not made wealthy, nor did he expect to become so. Doctors and nurses should be well paid, but not enriched, by their professional practice. At age four my son was asked what his parents did for a living. He replied that his mother was a lawyer and worked for money, while his father was a doctor who took care of sick people. That distinction, which made sense to a four-year-old, should inform every part of the health-care delivery system today.

Over my many years as a public-health consultant, I was paid well to provide expert testimony. For example, after I left Nevada and joined the faculty at the National Jewish Center in Denver Colorado, toward the end of one of the higher-profile cases with which I was associated, my deposition was taken by a couple dozen lawyers over about a two-week period of time, in two installments. My fees for preparing and rendering this sworn testimony were enough to pay for much of the cost of my oldest child's first year at an Ivy League university.

I had much to say about the case, which involved health problems related to the Polk County Courthouse. I worked with several hundred occupants of that problem building for a number of years, personally conducting extensive clinical and epidemiologic studies about the building-related illnesses that had occurred. Some of this data has been published and can be reviewed by the interested reader.[12]

Briefly stated, this ten-story building opened just after construction with marked moisture-incursion problems and consequent mold growth. There were rooms in the building where the mold grew carpet-thick and multicolored on the walls. The county maintenance crews would sandblast the mold off the walls while the clerical staff of the courts sat at their desks in the same room.

This problem went on for two years until the office of the prosecuting attorney moved out of the building and threatened to stop appearing in any of the courtrooms until the problem was fixed, thus threatening to shut down the criminal justice system in the county. Many occupants of the building were ill with respiratory symptoms such as cough, wheezing, and shortness of breath. These people were naturally frightened.

Additionally, they were persuaded that the county administration didn't care at all about the health problems they'd developed. They were deeply suspicious that I'd been hired by the administration to downplay the health problems so the county could get on with a "cheap" fix for the building problems. Having discovered this latent feeling of hostility, I made it a practice to hold an open meeting with the building occupants each time I ventured to Bartow, the town where the courthouse was situated.

My first such meeting occurred at the end of my first trip to Bartow, which lasted about ten days. During that sojourn, I'd interviewed several dozen building occupants and concluded that an observational epidemiologic study of the entire population was warranted. Accordingly, written questionnaires (about twenty pages long, as I remember) were prepared for all the occupants of the courthouse and a neighboring county structure (to be used as a comparison population)—a total of about one thousand persons. We achieved well over 90 percent participation in the questionnaire. The people who attended the open meeting had all answered the questions. They were furious about many of the questions and about things a few of them felt should have been on the questionnaire but weren't.

Public-health science is often derived in exactly that kind of heated environment, with strong opinions already belching from a furnace of fomenting anxiety. The questionnaire data documented a high likelihood of allergic respiratory disease, such as asthma, among those with substantial mold exposure in the problem building. Follow-up clinical evaluations of selected sick-building occupants documented the occurrence of serious allergic disease of the chest. These findings substantially changed the building renovation project. The original cost of construction had been about $12 million. The county expected a far lower cost to renovate and had actually turned down a $4 million offer from a Hollywood production company asking to use the building during a film project, because too much destruction of the existing structure would've been incidental to the filming.

Ultimately, as I recall, something approaching $30 million was spent on the building project. For a time, I believe I was viewed as the cause of much of this excess cost, and the project chief tried to have me replaced with a physician more "friendly" to a less expensive renovation. I was asked to present myself before the county commission to answer their concerns about the project.

During that hearing, dozens of building occupants, by then persuaded by the clinical and epidemiologic evidence I had accumulated, testified to the commissioners that they would not reenter the renovated courthouse unless Dr. Jarvis certified it was safe to do so. While I was paid well for all the work I did on that case, money couldn't buy the sense of purpose and peace I received from persistently applying good public health and clinical science to a difficult situation.

I've always tried to remain true to those principles, believing that most people can eventually understand good science when it's presented to them. I believe the rule of law is only possible when the majority seeks good information and applies it in pursuit of the common good. Professional fees should be a byproduct of applying useful science, not the principle reason for participation.

In Nevada, however, I'd seen how money disrupted the rule of law on several occasions when I encountered the remarkable power of the medical industrial complex. During the legislative session just prior to my arrival as the state health officer, the Nevada legislature passed a bill requiring the Nevada Division of Health to regulate specialized and expensive hospital services, such as newborn intensive care, organ transplantation, burn care, open heart surgery, and trauma care.

It was my understanding that this legislation had come about in part because Nevada's hospitals were thought to be the most expensive in the nation on a per-bed/-day basis. I'd personally experienced this excess cost just after arriving in Nevada, when my wife delivered our fourth child in Reno a few months after we moved there.

At the time, we were still carrying health insurance with my Utah employer. The billed charges for the hospital, obstetrician, and anesthesiologist were about twice the usual and customary fees for the same services in Utah. This was despite the fact that as soon as we moved to Reno and became acquainted with the medical community there, we were directly informed by pediatricians that if any problems occurred during the pregnancy, we should immediately return to Utah for the delivery since newborn intensive care in Reno was very substandard.

As I further explored the medical community in Nevada, I discovered that many more of the sophisticated services I'd been accustomed to having for my patients in Utah were not as good—or simply not available—in Nevada. Why should a demonstrably poorer quality health-care system cost almost twice as much as the higher quality care delivered next door in Utah?

In fact, poor quality health care that is inefficiently financed will always cost more than care delivered in a better system. This is the most ignominious flaw of the American health-care delivery system. We Americans are given poor quality care in our clinics, operating rooms, emergency rooms, hospitals, nursing homes, intensive care units, and in every other health-care setting. American health-care delivery does the right thing for the patient, delivers the correct medication or the needed service, about half the time.

Too many American patients have surgeries and other interventions that are not clinically indicated and have little or no chance of improving patient health (remember the gall bladder operation in Fallon, Nevada, and the hysterectomy in Salt Lake City, Utah?) And in the process of delivering medical care, patients are injured far too often. These three types of poor-quality care cost a fortune, because in health care, when the patient's status is worse, more care is required. You can't simply throw the mistakes away. Meanwhile, payments for these services are made unnecessarily complicated by the health-insurance business model. Providers of care have entire rooms full of billing agents trying to get the institution paid. Insurers have more rooms full of claims processors whose job it is to find fault with every billing and to delay or deny payment. Nevada's poorer quality care was, therefore, directly related to why the care cost so much more than in Utah. And as to inefficiency in the health financing sector, well, my duties as state health officer opened my eyes.

One of the onerous duties I had as state health officer was to share the regulation of all HMOs (health maintenance organizations) with the Nevada commissioner of insurance. The insurance commissioner was required to regulate the business practices of the HMOs, all of which at that time were for-profit (and presumably still are). This meant assuring, by way of compliance regulation, that the individual HMO would have enough funds to meet all potential financial obligations to those persons in Nevada who had purchased a health plan from the HMO.

My job, according to Nevada statute, was to make sure each HMO had an adequate network of health-care facilities and professionals to serve the medical needs of each plan member. On my first day as the Nevada state health officer (along with that infamous typhoid fever report), I was met with several large volumes of files concerning an application of the state's largest HMO, Health Plan of Nevada. They wanted to expand their operations from the Las Vegas area in Southern Nevada to Reno and other portions of Northern Nevada.

I spent hours reviewing contracts HPN had arranged with various medical groups in Northern Nevada, including most physician specialties, various hospitals, and other kinds of care, such as physical therapy. Meanwhile, HPN sent its chief government liaison officer to see me. She wanted to know how I planned to proceed with their application. They recognized they didn't have any orthopedic surgeons on contract in Northern Nevada, and she explained the reason: none of the orthopedic surgeons in Reno would agree to the contract terms offered by HPN.

She was worried I might allow the recalcitrance of a few orthopedic surgeons to hold the HPN application hostage. In response, I explained that the state board of health ultimately had the authority to approve or deny the application and that I would put the question about the orthopedic-care contract to them. However, I asked her to provide a letter to the file that guaranteed that any HPN member in Northern Nevada who needed orthopedic care would have access to and financing for the care as needed. With that letter in hand, I reported the application to the board favorably, and the board approved it.

A few months later, I began receiving complaints about HPN from doctors in Northern Nevada. Apparently, the ear, nose, and throat group that had originally agreed to provide services for HPN members under contract decided to leave the HPN network. In response, HPN arranged for an ENT physician from their Southern Nevada group to come once each month to Reno to see HPN patients in consultation.

This had not proven adequate for the urgent care ENT problems (bloody noses, punctured ear drums, etc.) that sometimes occurred. In addition to being unable to get ENT care for their HPN patients, physicians under contract with HPN in Northern Nevada were complaining about the business practices of the organization. The physicians made allegations about claims not being paid, or being down categorized, or about payments delayed for many months.

Eventually, the Nevada insurance commissioner asked me to join him in holding a public hearing about these complaints concerning HPN business practices in Northern Nevada. We rented the city council chambers in Reno and invited any interested parties to come and present testimony. It turned into an acrimonious, hours-long debacle from which I doubted any good could be extracted. Soon after, I received an anonymous complaint that a newborn delivered during a weekend in Carson City had not received any medical attention after its birth prior to its discharge home.

The mother was an HPN member and had been attended during labor and delivery by an HPN contracted obstetrician, but apparently HPN hadn't arranged for pediatric services at the hospital during that particular weekend. This was a clear violation of the regulatory requirements for an HMO. The statute provided for fines and other administrative penalties to be adjudicated by the Nevada Board of Health. Consequently, I documented the violation and noticed an emergency change to the upcoming board agenda. I presented the evidence to the board and asked it to fine HPN (a few thousand dollars was the limit of the fine, as I recall). To my surprise, the board refused to levy the penalty, even though they agreed the violation had occurred. They ordered me to check regularly on the status of services to be sure the same kind of problem didn't recur.

I felt like I was being punished. I had no staff or budget for HMO supervision. Every hour I spent on HMO regulation seemed both ineffective in getting better quality care delivered to Nevadans and a loss to other, more traditional public-health programs I could be supporting.

HPN staff were frequently on the phone or in my office trying to persuade me that I could ignore complaints. I was even invited to visit their office in Las Vegas to meet the CEO (a physician trained in cardiology who'd left medical practice to make tens of millions of dollars selling health plans) and work out our differences. We met in the boardroom on the top floor of a building full of HPN employees. From that room, we had an expansive view in all directions: Mount Charleston to the west, the Las Vegas Strip to the south, Sunrise Mountain to the east. The room was solid oak, plush, and beautiful. There were fifteen high-level executives around the table with their CEO, and then there was me.

It was intended to be intimidating, but it clearly demonstrated that the problems HPN was having paying for and delivering services in Northern Nevada had nothing to do with a lack of funds. It had to do with a business model that was, first and foremost, all about how to make as much money as possible. Patient care was of lesser (if any) significance. Inefficiencies in managing claims, such as delaying payment to physicians, were merely business practices intended to make more money for HPN, no matter what consequences ensued for patients.

The CEO of HPN was fond of saying that for-profit health-care companies like his were better for patients than nonprofit firms because the for-profit businesses were accountable to investors, while nonprofits had no such accountability. It's true that the managers of for-profit companies have a fiduciary duty to the stockholders to make as much money as possible. But they have no fiduciary relationship with patients. In fact, HPN principally made money by *not* paying for health care. As far as I know, HPN, or Sierra Health Services, as I believe it is now called, is still making millions of dollars for its investors.

At about that same time, Humana decided to organize its first Nevada HMO. Again, I received many volumes of contract documents I had to review in advance of a Nevada Board of Health meeting. As I met with the Humana representatives, as per my usual approach to the upcoming board meeting, I didn't indicate what my recommendation to the board might be. I felt I had a duty to inform the board first, in open meeting, as required by state statute, about the results of my investigation.

I suppose not knowing how their application might be handled made the Humana representatives nervous. On the day of the board hearing, as I arrived at the venue for the meeting, I met the lead Humana executive. He approached me as I was assembling my notes in preparation for the meeting and told me point blank that if I would agree to report his application favorably, he promised to hire me at a six-figure salary (a large salary for the time) as the first medical director of the HMO. Though I had by then fielded many threats to my job, I'd not yet been offered a job as inducement to use my office of public trust selectively. I'd had many offers of meals, gratuities, favors, gifts, etc., all of which had been presented away from the public eye. Certainly never just as a public hearing was about to convene.

The chief administrative officer of the Nevada Health Division to whom I submitted my receipts for travel and other expenses made it clear from my first day at the health division that I was to always pay for my own meals and never accept gifts. So the routine gratuities were easy enough to forgo. They bounced off me like the threats to my job. But I was dumbfounded by the blatant bribe attempt at the board of health meeting.

I told the Humana representative to take his seat and ignored him. I went ahead and did what I'd planned to do, which was offer a favorable report about the Humana application to the board of health. Over the years since then, I've come to know that this is routine practice in the medical industrial complex.

Who can forget Billy Tauzin, the Louisiana congressman who helped get Medicare Part D passed in the form most favorable to the drug industry, only to resign Congress and accept appointment as the chief lobbyist for Big Pharma at $2 million per year?

He eventually received a salary of $11.6 million in 2010, making him the highest paid health lobbyist at the time. It's often said that one gets what one pays for. In health care, we get what the corporate health lobby pays for us to receive. Why would Humana offer to double my salary without even looking at my qualifications for the job? And why did Big Pharma pay Mr. Tauzin up to $50 million over a decade of employment? Obviously because the medical industrial complex knows how important the government revenue streams are to health care, and they want people with inside experience in government to show the way in keeping those revenue streams flowing.

Health-care corporations love to talk about the private market, but they feed at the public trough like no other sector of the economy. In Utah, the director of the health department recently resigned (summer 2015) to take a job running a for-profit HMO that principally does business with the Utah Medicaid program—the same program he personally supervised while serving as an executive in state government. This kind of revolving door into high-paid health-care sector jobs happens so routinely no one even reports about it anymore.

In response to the aforementioned legislation just prior to my arrival in the Silver State, the Nevada Health Division made a remarkable effort, led primarily by Larry Matheis, to put into regulation how trauma services were to be delivered. After the board of health passed these regulations, a request for proposals was published. Larry and I hoped that a number of hospitals in Las Vegas (and perhaps one or two in Reno) would respond to the RFP and compete for the highest level designation as a trauma center.

We were to be disappointed. Only one hospital in Las Vegas responded. Unfortunately, when we assembled a team of experts to review that hospital's proposal for trauma care, we discovered that the facility failed to meet the level of care required by our newly passed regulations. Thus, we found ourselves in a political predicament. The Nevada legislature expected the Nevada Division of Health to designate a high-level trauma center in Las Vegas, we'd passed regulations expecting such a designation to occur, and then the only hospital that had opted to apply had failed to meet the standards set. Embarrassing.

There was a hospital in Las Vegas, however, which I'm sure would have passed muster with the trauma review. At that time, the hospital was owned by Humana. In fact, it was said to be the most profitable hospital in the Humana system nationwide. One day soon after the sole applicant hospital failed its review for the high-level trauma center designation, I happened to have business at the Humana hospital and ran into the CEO. I used the chance meeting as an opportunity to ask him about his choice to not apply for the trauma-center designation.

First I asked him if it was true that the presidential advance team consistently chose his hospital as the place they would bring President Reagan if he were to be injured. (President Reagan was often in state because he was trying to support the reelection efforts of Senator Chic Hecht, in vain, as it turned out.)

The CEO confirmed that his hospital was the trauma center of choice for the White House advance team. Then I reminded him we'd recently published a request for proposals for trauma care in Southern Nevada and hadn't received a bid from him, which led to the awkward situation of having a statutory requirement for regulated trauma care but no applicants worthy of the designation. Why, I asked, had he not responded to the RFP? I assured him that trauma care good enough for President Reagan was very likely optimal for residents of Southern Nevada.

His response was remarkably candid. He pointed out that the Nevada Division of Health had licensed his hospital for 450 beds (I believe that number to be correct but can't verify this assertion). However, he routinely staffed the hospital for far fewer patients, maybe as few as 350 active beds. He then stated that if the staffed hospital beds were full and a patient arrived at the ER needing hospital admission, his staff made a judgment call. If the ER patient had adequate means to pay for hospitalization, his staff called in additional nurses, thus staffing up to a higher number of beds, and admitted the patient. On the other hand, if his staff were convinced the ER patient didn't have the means to pay for hospitalization, his staff informed the patient there were no available beds and transfer to another facility would be necessary. The CEO then noted that the trauma regulations as written and passed by the Nevada Board of Health required the hospital with the highest level trauma care designation to take all emergency patients with trauma—without regard to ability to pay.

This would circumvent the judgment calls of his staff about admitting ER patients, and that, he could not allow. He made it clear he was in the business of making money, not providing Southern Nevadans with trauma care. This was another surreal moment for me in Nevada. But it felt more threatening than the purple world of microbiological disease.

Be clear about the for-profit, market-based health-care delivery system we have allowed to flourish in our country. It's designed to make as much money as possible—not provide the best health care possible. One cannot maximize profits *and* optimize care. In the United States, we have the most profitable health-care system in the world. And, consequently, we have the worst health-care quality in the first world, at the highest price.

I had similar purple-world experiences while trying to regulate open-heart surgery care and neonatal intensive care in Nevada hospitals. For both kinds of care, I received assistance from Nevada physicians who knew from professional experience how to deliver high-quality care. Guidelines for the delivery of open-heart surgery care had been published by the American College of Surgery. We adapted those guidelines into a regulatory format and published the draft regulations for public comment. Likewise, the draft regulations for neonatal intensive care consisted of an adaptation of the guidelines published by the combined efforts of the American Academy of Pediatrics and the American College of Obstetrics and Gynecology. These draft guidelines were also put out for public comment throughout Nevada. For both sets of drafted regulations, the problems came from Reno.

In that relatively modest-sized city, there were two hospitals that both hoped to deliver these services. In the case of open-heart surgery, there were not enough cases per year to justify designating two institutions. Only one hospital would qualify. The hospital that didn't receive the open-heart surgery designation sued the state of Nevada. The attorney general in Nevada chose not to oppose the lawsuit, effectively killing the regulations.

These same two hospitals didn't openly fight over neonatal intensive care. Rather, they entered into a joint operating agreement. They hired one group of doctors to be the clinicians in the two hospitals, each of which had a unit designated as newborn intensive care. Sick newborns delivered in either hospital would be admitted to the birthing hospital's newborn intensive care unit (NICU). In reality, this was a pretense of high-level neonatal care delivery with the expectation that both hospitals would be paid as if they were competently caring for newborns.

For instance, the doctor on call for sick newborns could not be in both hospitals at once. Most of the physicians delivering this care were not trained in neonatology. Apparently, the two hospitals were saving money by hiring fewer and less well-trained physicians, among several other shortcuts. They jointly asked the state for a variance from the neonatal care regulations, allowing them to continue to deliver substandard care. The mortality rate for sick newborns was twice as high in Reno as it was in Las Vegas. This is the sickening purple world of the American way of doing health-care business. They received their variance as soon as I resigned from my duties as state health officer and was no longer at the Nevada Board of Health meetings to oppose them.

As part of the faculty of National Jewish Hospital in Denver, a facility which specialized in the care of respiratory diseases, I was part of a very high-quality practice that received referrals from all over the United States of patients with the most challenging lung diseases.

Not infrequently, patients would come to see me in the clinic directly after landing at the Denver airport. On one such occasion, a man with serious black-lung disease arrived in Denver from Kentucky the day of his initial clinic visit with me. When I saw him in the outpatient setting a few hours after his flight touched down at Denver's altitude, I noticed he was struggling to breathe and was blue about his lips. I concluded he needed to be admitted to the inpatient part of National Jewish Hospital and wrote the appropriate orders.

I left the clinic for fifteen minutes and returned to find him getting sicker but still sitting in the waiting room. I immediately asked the nurse why he hadn't been taken to his hospital room, and she replied that the business office of the hospital wouldn't allow the transfer to occur because he had prior approval for an outpatient evaluation, not an inpatient admission.

When business decisions supersede the emergent needs of patients, even at the hospital that prides itself on being the best of its kind in treating lung disease, the purple world in health care can make even one's best efforts as a physician become insignificant. So I gave up trying. I quit practicing clinical medicine and devoted myself professionally to public policy and consulting.

At the time I left Utah and moved my family to Arlington, Virginia, to start my public-health career, I chose to stop doing obstetrical care, though I continued to work part-time as a family physician. But my reasons for discontinuing obstetrical practice were very different from my reasons for ceasing to provide clinical care at all. Just before I moved from Utah, I had two experiences with critical care wherein I had cause to question whether I was as good at obstetrical and neonatal services as any other available provider.

The first experience came at the end of what appeared to be a normal labor and delivery. Once I cut the umbilical cord and turned to hand the baby over to the nurse, my maternal patient began rapidly bleeding from a vaginal source. In fact, she was exsanguinating. I had only moments to discover the source of the bleeding and staunch it, or she would die. The lacerations may have happened due to my decision to use forceps during the delivery, but I couldn't be sure—lacerations can happen without the use of instruments.

Using a long-handled clamp, I did find deep bilateral cervical lacerations and was able to stop the bleeding. The repair of the lacerations was well beyond my skill set. I asked for the gynecologist on-call to come, and I spent four hours assisting him with the necessary surgery.

The other critical moment of care also came during what had been a routine obstetrical experience. My maternal patient had been scheduled for a C-section at full-term. I'd referred her to an obstetrician for the surgery because I didn't include C-sections in my practice. I attended the delivery in order to care for the baby. Everything went well until I was handed the infant, who wasn't breathing. Again, I had only moments to make a difference. Ultimately, just as I was preparing to intubate the baby, he took a deep breath and began to cry.

These two episodes, which both happened during the same on-call weekend, caused me to consider whether I was really as good at delivering care in critical moments as my patients deserved. Both patients survived, and my interventions had been adequate, but I concluded that there were better trained doctors available. I decided to leave the practice of obstetrics and neonatal care to them.

Chapter Ten

Red and Blue Health Policy Proposals—
One and the Same

SINCE LEAVING NEVADA, and then leaving clinical practice in Colorado, I've tried to get a seat at the tables at which health policy is made. I've tried lobbying legislators, organizing coalitions, joining movements for health-system reform, and accepted countless invitations to speak or debate about the topic. I started a nonprofit organization, the Utah Health Policy Project, and solicited tens of thousands of dollars in donations so that there could be a credible source of health-policy information available to the public in Utah. We studied every issue, followed every federal and Utah bill, wrote numerous opinion pieces, tracked down every reporter on the health beat, applied to be on every radio talk show, and generally made a nuisance of ourselves about health policy. I was invited into a select few back rooms (which in Utah are not filled with smoke), but once there, found I had little influence on the outcome of the discussion.

I decided to run for the legislature in 2006. I won a hotly contested race for the Republican nomination for a state senate seat in a decidedly Democrat Salt Lake City district. My campaign was favored by the endorsement of the editors of the *Salt Lake Tribune,* the largest "independent" newspaper in Utah, because, they said, I brought fresh ideas about health-system reform into electoral politics.

Those in the Republican Party who offered me advice—and there were several—insisted I solicit campaign donations from corporate power players in the state. However, the big problem for me was that the biggest corporate donors to candidates were from the health-care sector (this was, and is, especially true for candidates at the federal level), none of whom liked my fresh ideas about health-system reform. Most corporate donors refused to meet with me. They knew I was unlikely to win and were not interested in working with someone who wasn't likely to hold elected office. Too often, voters also choose candidates—not based upon what good they might accomplish—but on the often-arbitrary determination of electability. So I contented myself with campaign donations from family and friends, leading to a campaign fund less than half the size of my Democrat opponent in the general election.

I was not elected. I lost and not mostly because I didn't have enough money to fund a viable campaign. I lost because of voter apathy and partisanship. If all the registered Republicans in the district had showed up to vote and had chosen to vote for me, I may have eked out a victory. But voter participation is remarkably low in our republic. Those who did vote didn't make an effort to understand anything about the candidates except their political party. My opponent received enough straight-party votes to win the election. A straight-party vote is an option any Utah voter can exercise on the first page of the ballot. Rather than marking the ballot with a specific candidate for each race, the straight-party voter simply marks the party choice on the first page and skips thinking about or even knowing the various candidates.

I went door to door in every precinct in the district. I mailed literature to every voting household several times. I attended and did well at every debate and candidate event. I had a campaign website and was the first legislative candidate in Utah to regularly podcast from the campaign trail. None of it mattered. Most of the few voters who bothered to exercise their franchise had predetermined a partisan basis for how to cast their ballot. Never mind health-system reform.

Upsets do occur in politics, though rarely. My good friend Bill Orton, a Democrat, represented the most Republican congressional district in Utah, probably in the nation, for three terms in the 1990s. Before his untimely death a few years ago, we were neighbors in Salt Lake City. I met him while he was running for governor and did my best to help his campaign. And he assisted me with my state senate race. During my uphill battle, I asked him how he'd managed to win office with such a heavy partisan bias against him. He explained that no Democrat had wanted the nomination for that congressional seat, so he'd run unopposed in the Democratic Party. Meanwhile, three Republicans were acrimoniously slugging it out for their nomination. The Republicans were holding a series of debates all over the district, mostly in very rural communities. Not having anything else to do, he asked each of the three if they would allow him to join them at their debates. His modest proposal was accepted, surprisingly, and he began traveling the district. He'd arrive a day or two before each debate and spend the time shadowing key people in each town as they went about their rural business.

He used the time and conversation to discover what those people were thinking. During each debate, he simply repeated to the audience what their community leaders had stated to him. Meanwhile, the Republican candidates were busy hacking away at each other, weakening the eventual nominee. Bill Orton won his first race because he told the electorate, those who were paying attention, what they wanted to hear, while the Republicans were snarling at each other.

Virtually all campaigns consist of having politicians tell the electorate what they want to hear, except not using the homespun methods of Bill Orton's first race. Candidates are schooled in the art of staying on message. I was often told as a candidate that I should never answer the questions posed to me. Instead, my campaign manager told me what she thought the particular audience of the day would want to hear and insisted that no matter what the question was, I was to stick to the talking points she provided. (I made a terrible politician because I couldn't break the habit of trying to honestly answer each question.)

Well-funded candidates take advantage of modern polling and other market research. They know what is on the minds of the people because they've paid experts to find out. Good politicians (the ones who get elected and then reelected) find out what the message is and then stick to the message. And they get their message out with the now-familiar uses of the media—either through paid advertising or arranging newsworthy events that get "covered."

For example, President Obama knew from polling that Americans were worried about whether health-system reform would allow them to choose their own doctors. So he stayed on that message: if you like your doctor, you can keep your doctor. President Trump did the same thing. He repeatedly told the electorate they would be pleased with the health care he would arrange as president. He says what he knows people want to hear, never mind whether he endorses the concept or not. And never mind that President Obama had no intention of keeping his promise. He made his real bargain with the health-insurance industry before he was even sworn into office, at least according to *Frontline* on PBS. Republicans are no better. They get their health-care talking points from the medical industrial complex too.

Staying current with what the electorate wants to hear takes a lot of money. Polling is expensive. Market research is a sophisticated, time-consuming process. Opinions change rapidly, so polling must be continuous and careful. Getting the message out is also expensive. Paid media—billboards, TV, radio, social media, and now, less commonly, newspapers and mailers—requires big money.

I hired six billboards for my campaign for six weeks at a cost of about $20,000, which was more than a third of my campaign budget. This is why corporate campaign donations are so important to candidates. Candidates who get elected know that to win the next election, they'll need corporate political donations. If their electorate wants to hear something that's not favorable to a corporate donor, they may choose to tell the voters what they want to hear, but they'll never act on a message that will disrupt the donation stream. This is why Dean Daugherty taught me to never trust a politician. It is time for all Americans to learn that lesson. No matter how red or blue leaning you are, don't believe any politician, whichever "color" they may be. Media pundits are, by and large, extensions of this same colored approach to policy conversation. Don't believe them either. In fact, don't listen to the slamming back and forth that passes for political discourse and is so popular on radio and television.

We only have ourselves to blame for our do-nothing Congress and state legislatures. We the American people are the voters of apathy who often don't vote at all or vote while being uninformed. We dislike Congress, but we keep reelecting the same people to serve in Congress. Candidates today can count on that kind of apathy from most of the people casting ballots. The remaining minority are partisans—they will vote by party affiliation, right or wrong. Republican partisans allege they vote for values or cherished beliefs. Democrat partisans tend to favor facts and science. But don't be fooled. I've attended many political meetings, both Republican and Democrat, and have yet to hear any serious policy discussion among these partisans at all, whether driven by values or by facts.

The reason there isn't a dime's worth of difference between the health policies proposed by the two major American political parties is that their principle purpose is to elect politicians, not actually serve the people of the United States. To do that, they need large cash contributions. Those contributions come from corporate interests, especially from the health-care sector. We won't make a difference in our health policy until politicians are unelected because they fail to effectively change how American health care is delivered. If you want Congress to be different, elect different people to Congress. If you don't make the effort to change Congress, then stop whining about Obamacare or Trumpcare.

You are getting the health-care system you deserve.

Chapter Eleven

Obamacare, Trumpcare, and Beyond

EVERYTHING WRONG ABOUT American health care was made worse by the implementation of the Patient Protection and Affordable Care Act, better known as Obamacare. I knew it would happen before he even took office. Between the election and the inauguration, the Obama campaign encouraged all Americans to attend neighborhood meetings where we could talk with fellow citizens about what we hoped health-system reform might accomplish.

I went to the neighborhood meeting so that I could hear what my neighbors had to say. There, I found a roomful of people who actually trusted Mr. Obama. They told me I should give him a chance. I wish there had been a reason to allow their hopes to play out. I'm not a cynic who only sees the glass half empty. Nor am I a conservative crank who would rather the country fail than have a Democrat succeed. Let me also restate that I know the common Republican slogan concerning Obamacare, "repeal and replace," is patently bogus, as is amply demonstrated by Trumpcare.

What Republicans offer is no better than Obamacare. In fact, when speaking about health-system reform, I commonly state that there's not a dime's worth of difference between the two parties when it comes to their health-care policies, despite the partisan bickering between them. But I recognized what Obama was peddling because I'd seen it before.

Ten years before Obamacare passed, I published an opinion piece in the *Deseret News,* from which I take the following:

We Americans are on the horns of a health-care dilemma. We have the most expensive health care in the world. We are more heavily taxed for health care than the citizens of any other country, even more taxed [for health care] than countries with so-called socialized medicine.

And unlike those other countries, in addition to our taxes, we also pay out-of-pocket expenses for premiums, deductibles, copayments and employer contributions for health care, making our health-care expenses twice as high as those paid on average by people living in other industrialized countries. And for that expense, we get fewer physician visits per capita, fewer hospital bed days per capita, limited choice of physician, poorer overall health for our citizens, increased personal bankruptcies and, unlike any other industrialized country, millions of our fellow citizens (300,000 in Utah) have no health insurance at all. Our dilemma is that we shell out incredible sums for health care and get so little in return. What are we to do?

On Dec. 18, [2000], the Health Insurance Association, the American Hospital Association, the American Nurses Association and Families USA, among others, will stage a health-care summit in Salt Lake City to discuss the solution that they propose for our health-care dilemma. They've already announced the plan they're promoting. They want the American taxpayer to come up with more money to fund health care for the uninsured. Surely, they argue, during our current good times, the wealthiest nation in the world can come up with the money to fund health insurance for every citizen.

Let us not be taken in by the health insurance industry. Our health-care dilemma is not caused by underfunding health care. The American taxpayer is the world's most generous where health care is concerned. We do not need more revenues for health care; we need to carefully spend the revenues we already have. The health insurance industry generally keeps up to 30 percent of our premiums for profits, executive salaries and bureaucratic red tape. Of course they want us to spend more on health care, because the more money in the health care financing system, the higher their salaries and profits. No amount of increase in health care funding will be enough to cover all Americans as long as the private health insurance and managed care sector is allowed to divert money away from patient care and into bureaucracies and bank accounts.

The only solution to our health-care dilemma is to end the domination of health-care financing by profit-taking health businesses.[13]

It's remarkable to me how closely the bill that was passed ten years later in Congress followed the proposal I referenced in December 2000. Health-care business as usual in the United States is always about making more sales of health-care goods and services (including useless, wasteful services like health-insurance policies) than it is about actually taking care of patients. Obama was following the health-insurance industry script, just like Republicans are doing now that they own the White House and Congress.

Obamacare basically raised more federal revenues from American taxpayers in order to buy more health insurance for Americans. As such, Obamacare, like many of the so-called major health-policy initiatives passed by Congress over the years (for example Medicare, Medicaid, and CHIP) is about "coverage" and not really about care. Once again, our political leaders got the diagnosis wrong concerning what sickness plagues American health-care delivery. Or, as Trudy Lieberman put it in the July 2015 issue of *Harper's Magazine*: the "wrong prescription" to treat America's health-care ills. Here is some of what she said:

> The A.C.A. was sold to the public on the pledge of "afford-able, quality health care," ... [which] persuaded the public that the A.C.A. was a vehicle for delivering universal healthcare, similar to what citizens had in other industrialized nations. It was not. Instead, the A.C.A. was a canny restructuring of the American

health-care marketplace, one that delivered millions of new customers to insurance companies, created new payment mechanisms for hospitals, steered more business to pharmaceutical companies, and dictated expensive, high-tech solutions for a wide range of problems. . . .

. . . The Congressional Budget Office estimates that even under the A.C.A., there will be some 35 million Americans without health insurance. . . . Whatever the slogans suggested, the A.C.A. was never meant to include everyone.

Essentially, the law is a means-tested program, like food stamps or Medicaid. It offers people the chance to buy private insurance online through a state- or federally run exchange, and to receive a government subsidy to help them pay their premiums. It is primarily aimed at the poor and the nearly poor: this year, 87 percent of A.C.A. enrollees qualified to receive monthly subsidies averaging $263 per person (at least in the thirty-seven states with federally run exchanges). To its credit, the law also allowed sick people to buy insurance and more of the neediest Americans to qualify for Medicaid. . . .

And what of those middle-class Americans who were supposed to benefit from the law, and were promised that they could keep the policies and health providers they already had? They've already been hit with higher premiums and higher out-of-pocket costs—and people with top-of-the-line coverage from their employers will soon find those policies shrinking, thanks to a provision of the law that encourages companies to offer less-generous benefits.

It's bad enough that the A.C.A. is fattening up the health-care industry and hollowing out coverage for the middle class. Even worse, the law is accelerating what I call the Great Cost Shift, which transfers the growing price of medical care to patients themselves through high deductibles, coinsurance (the patient's share of the cost for a specific service, calculated as a percentage), copayments (a set fee paid for a specific service), and limited provider networks (which sometimes offer so little choice that patients end up seeking out-of-network care and paying on their own). What was once good, comprehensive insurance for a sizable number of Americans is being reduced to coverage for only the most serious, and most expensive, of illnesses. Even fifteen years ago, families paid minimal deductibles of $150 or $200 and copays of $5 or $10, or none at all. Now, a family lucky enough to afford a policy in the first place may face out-of-pocket expenses for coinsurance, deductibles, and copays as high as $13,200 before its insurer kicks in. Of course, these out-of-pocket caps can be adjusted by the insurer every year, within limits set by the government, and there are no caps at all for out-of-network services, which means that some providers charge whatever the market will bear. In the post-A.C.A. era, you can be insured but have little or no coverage for what you actually need.[14]

Trumpcare will make all of these problems worse.

What was it like to be an American seeking health care after the passage of Obamacare? For my family, with insurance through my spouse's employment as a senior partner in a major national law firm, little changed. When we were sick or injured (and as we age, that happens more frequently), we expected to pay very high out-of-pocket costs for the care we needed. Our combined income gave us flexibility, however, and so we chose our own physicians, whether in or out of network, and paid for it.

The vast majority of Americans have not been able to afford for themselves the kind of care we have. As a physician, I'm able to make decisions for myself and my family that reduce our reliance on the kindness of strangers within the health-care delivery system. I commonly stay at the bedside of my hospitalized relatives and render needed assistance, including insisting with hospital staff that timely nursing is provided. I know that profit margins have diminished bedside care in modern American hospitals. In fact, the ability to help my family is one of the reasons I chose to enter the medical profession.

In college, while newly married, I experienced the neglect of health professionals so common in American health care. Just as I was making the decision whether to accept a scholarship to law school or a place in medical school, my first child was born. We were at Brigham Young University in Provo, Utah; therefore, we lived among many hundreds of young couples beginning their families. The OB had more patients than he should have been allowed. Most were young and healthy, so they tended to do well despite his lack of proper attendance. My wife was in labor for seventy-two hours before delivering, and the OB came in only at the very last second. Not once did he examine her throughout her protracted labor, which constitutes great neglect. Things could've easily turned out much worse than they did. After that, I was determined that I'd never leave my wife, children, and grandchildren so vulnerable again.

I learned later while receiving OB training, how badly performing the doctor had been. But his care was the standard at Utah Valley Hospital at that time. As a lay person, I had no way of making an impact on that care situation. I've found, however, that as a doctor, I can always get a response from care providers now.

Even with that resolve, my training as a doctor, and my interest in health policy, I've encountered very difficult moments while trying to troubleshoot my family's health care. When one of my close family members required expensive orthopedic surgery available from only two providers in our hometown, our health insurer informed us that neither physician was "in network" for our plan. I inquired about how much our plan would pay for the needed surgery but initially received no answer. So I asked the hospital and doctor how much the procedure would cost but again received no answer.

We resolved the situation by relying on my contacts as a physician within the medical network to gain a sympathetic hearing of our problem by the providers while my spouse used her clout as a senior law partner to induce a more helpful approach by her firm's health insurer. Our combined professional clout made a huge difference. But the vast majority of Americans would have been left out in the health-care wilderness described by Ms. Lieberman—insured but with little or no coverage.

Or, perhaps, more likely, Americans are experiencing a health-care system that has no interest in providing any help at all, such as is true for another family I know; I'll call them the Simons. Fred Simon is a forty-two-year-old who works in construction. He has been married for thirteen years to Angela, who is thirty-three years old and currently works from home while taking care of her three young children. Angela was a manager for a local advertising company, at which job she had a health benefit (monthly cost of $800 paid half and half by herself and her employer) for the only time in her adult life. Months after Obamacare passed, she was laid off, which she believes was not coincidental. Angela has had asthma since age three, always well-controlled on one or two medications. Fred has no pre-existing conditions. The couple sought replacement health insurance (he has no possibility of a health benefit at his work) but found the $1,000-per-month premium and crazy out-of-pocket costs to be too expensive.

They were uninsured for their most recent pregnancy, labor, and delivery. Shopping among obstetrical offices did them no good because no one was willing to disclose a price for the service. They eventually chose a midwife for the delivery because she was willing to offer a firm price for her services. The couple had no contingency plans to pay for a complicated delivery or sick newborn, neither of which, fortunately, occurred. During the much-ballyhooed rollout of the Obamacare website, Angela made a major effort to find a health-insurance policy for her family. She found herself doubting the security of the website. She was frustrated by the difficulty of navigating the options. She was unable to make changes to her profile and choices. The help function was, well, not helpful. She was offered a discount on the premium but with the caveat that she'd be back-billed if, in fact, the family's income came in higher than expected.

Ultimately, she decided it was better to pay the Obamacare penalty (or was it tax?) than buy the policy, because at least that cost of the decision was knowable. The family has purchased a membership in a kind of medical co-op service for $100 per month plus a $10 copay per visit. With this, they receive essential primary-care services, including acute illness and injury care (one daughter's broken nose was handled, for instance, as have been ear infections and flu). Vaccines are not provided, but the family receives these at a public-health clinic. The membership will not cover catastrophic illness and injury, but Angela has a friend who did buy insurance yet nonetheless found that an ER visit was not covered anyway. So, philosophically, they believe themselves better off saving the $12,000-per-year premium and hoping for good health.

One problem is that their co-op does not cover medications, so Angela's asthma medication cost of $250 per month is stressing the family budget. So instead of doing the prescribed two puffs of medication twice a day, Angela takes one puff a day, or even less often.

I ask you, is this a health-care system you and all Americans are proud to support? We have rising death rates due to asthma in the United States during a time when better asthma treatments are available than has ever been the case. Yet here in the United States, where the clinical science to study the problem of asthma was conducted at the expense of the tax-payer, there are millions of taxpayers who can't afford to have asthma treatment. After wanting to give Obama his chance to show us he would come through for us, why did my neighbors vote to keep him in office another four years even though Obamacare is manifestly such a failure? Once Trumpcare fulfills its promise of being even worse than Obamacare, will Trump be reelected?

How bad did Obamacare fail? Listen to how Trudy Lieberman put it in the previously cited *Harper's Magazine* article:

> An affordability crisis is looming. Last fall, The Common-wealth Fund found that almost half of all insured adults with incomes of $23,000 or less delayed or skipped care because of high cost-sharing expenses, regardless of which kind of insurance they had. In a December [2014] *New York Times*/CBS News poll, 46 percent of respondents described health-care costs as a hard-ship, up from 36 percent the previous year. . . .
>
> . . . The average deductible this year for bronze policies, the cheapest on the exchanges, is $5,181 for individuals and $10,545 for families. . . . The perversity of selling cheap government-subsidized policies to the poor, then sticking them with gigantic

out-of-pocket costs, can hardly be lost on the 2.6 million people who opted for bronze plans on exchanges this year. . . .

The pricing of premiums, too, calls into question a leading premise of the A.C.A. Caroline Pearson, a senior vice president at the consulting firm Avalere Health, concedes that premiums on the exchanges have so far "turned out to be lower than what policymakers expected. But that still doesn't make them affordable for people on limited incomes." Even for families with incomes between $40,000 and $80,000, she says, "the math doesn't work out." In other words, the subsidies diminish rapidly as income rises, meaning that even slightly wealthier Americans may find it hard to afford healthcare. This helps to explain why about 22 percent of those who signed up on the federal exchange in 2014 did not come back this year. Roughly a third of enrollees on the state exchanges also declined to renew their policies. It's possible that some of these Americans found coverage from employers, or from insurers selling policies outside the exchanges. But some surely gave up because they couldn't afford the premiums or the cost-sharing—they couldn't afford to be sick.[15]

Why did President Obama sign into law a bill with such empty promises? Why has Trump revealed legislation that is a mockery of his campaign promises? (And I have not even begun to detail how Obamacare worsened the federal debt, virtually all of which was due to unfunded future health-care obligations even before the passage of the Affordable Care Act.) Well, he signed it because there were those realizing massive benefits from Obamacare. They were arguing for exactly this kind of legislation a decade before the passage of Obamacare, when I wrote that opinion piece in the *Deseret News*. They are the same organizations who benefitted from the passage of Romneycare in Massachusetts in 2006 (which, of course, is not significantly different from Obamacare). In fact, whether Republicans or Democrats are the moving force behind health-care legislation, it's always these same entities who benefit. Who are they? Again, Trudy Lieberman:

The biggest winners, of course, are the insurance companies themselves—especially those that grew and consolidated over the past few decades. The law has handed them millions of new customers. Competition is unlikely to drive down costs; five big insurers now dominate the market, making it extremely difficult for newcomers to gain a toehold....

...In California, for example, four big carriers sell 94 percent of the policies on the exchanges. "Not only is there significant market concentration," said David Jones, the state's insurance commissioner, "but only three insurers are selling statewide." Throughout much of California, Jones told me, this lack of competition "has tremendous implications for price and choice."

As long as market competition is restricted and there is no rate regulation (which is the case in fifteen states), rates will go up, Jones warns....

The same battle is going on across the country, and the ultimate loser is almost always the consumer. As hospitals consolidate with one another and with physician groups, it's hard to count on competition to keep costs down. Massachusetts is the poster child in this respect....

Shouldn't Massachusetts, which pioneered A.C.A.-style insurance exchanges almost a decade ago, be leading the nation in the law's implementation? Instead, it has the highest per capita health costs in the country, and health-care spending accounts for almost half of the state's current budget. Premiums are still rising, especially for workers in small businesses, who have been pinched by double-digit rate increases in seven of the past ten years. (The reason is that Romneycare merged the insurance risk pool, combining individual consumers and small employers—in effect, small employers subsidize individuals.) "It is no surprise to us in Massachusetts that the shortcomings of the basic framework of the Affordable Care Act mean marketplace discrimination for small businesses and their employees," argued Jon Hurst, the president of the Retailers Association of Massachusetts, in the *Boston Globe*.[16]

Affordable, quality care was the empty promise of Obamacare. No patients were protected, and there was nothing affordable about the implementation of this legislation. Republican proposals to repeal and replace Obamacare were worse. Neither party offered anything useful to the American people about how to fix our health-system mess.

Every other first-world nation has done a better job with health-care policy than has our nation. In Europe and Asia, health care is less costly, taxpayers pay lower health-care taxes, and patients have better access to the full range of health-care services, from primary care to highly intense hospitalization, than do Americans.

I did not start my professional life believing that American health care was a failing enterprise. But my experience has shocked me, driven me out of clinical care, and changed my approach to health-care reform. I hope what I've said in this book about my experience has shocked you, gentle reader, as well.

The American health-care system is the ultimate purple world. It costs twice as much to get health care in the United States, on a comparable basis, as it does to be treated in any other first-world nation. We're repeatedly told by both red and blue politicians that these high costs are because Americans have the best health-care system and being the best costs more. Further, both red and blue politicians want us to believe that a highly profitable, "marketized" health-care system is best because anything else would be socialized medicine, which would obviously be bad (fear-mongering at its worst).

This rhetoric is written in the boardrooms of big-health businesses that deliver talking points to the tongues of our politicians while massive political donations are changing hands. Meanwhile, a planeload of American patients dies from preventable injury in hospitals every other week, and American health care is the least able to concentrate clinical science to prevent death among all first-world health-care delivery systems. The purple world of American health care boils down to this: we pay more for care and get less care, but we do have the world's most profitable health-care corporations. Obamacare made this worse, not better, and Trumpcare aggravates the situation again.

The remedy for the purple world of American health care is, ironically, the creation of a politically purple nation. This is heavy political lifting. By that, I mean our nation must become less a collection of automatic red and blue states and more a community without a partisan predilection, in a fashion not unlike the surprising fall of the blue wall in the upper Midwest in November 2016. We must have more purple states, congressional districts, and legislative districts, meaning more places where elections are always contested, where the outcome is unpredictable and predicated upon sincerely held values and solidly observed facts, and where voters don't mind switching back and forth between parties. We must stop trusting the political class—all of them—no matter whether they be our preferred color or the alternative. Americans must stop voting by party and instead choose to vote by results.

Thomas Friedman wrote in the *New York Times* in January 2016[17] that Americans should adopt a bipartisan extremism in coming elections. They should look for leaders who could be honest with the electorate about complex issues instead of approaching everything as their political party dictated. The appeal of a leader who could combine the best ideas of each party would change the face of American politics and speak to the majority of Americans, who aren't rank-and-file versions of a Republican or Democrat.

Red-state citizens lean conservative and tend to couch their arguments in terms of the values and principles they hold or defend, like free markets, balanced budgets, and individual responsibility. Blue-state voters are often persuaded by facts, like how poverty affects people, or how programs can improve opportunity, or how every patient needs cancer screening. Yet when reds and blues have each most recently actually proposed and passed a health-care policy, they both proposed the same idea, which idea (whether Obamacare or Romneycare or Trumpcare) fails the patient while maximizing health-care profits. Because I have lobbied for real health-system change with elected officials from both parties, I know from personal experience that both sides know and use the talking points developed by the medical industrial complex. Yet, with no real policy differences, they still insist that only they have the people's best interests in view while demonizing the other side.

When health-care reform devolves into this kind of an ideological standoff, the public debate becomes acrimonious as even minor compromises become unacceptable and all possible common ground becomes an alleged slippery slope. Under these conditions, lobbyists can use political access to frame the debate for each side according to partisanship while continuing to protect their own interests. Ultimately, nobody is sincere or believable to the public and everything becomes a conspiracy. Meanwhile, the average citizen who has no dog in the ideological catfight often chooses to disengage, which only aggravates the problem by creating more elbow room for the ideologues.

The truth is that both facts and values matter to all of us. I love both the values of biblical living and the facts of public-health science. Together, these two ways of approaching public policy can fashion a first-rate US health-care system. Organizing the policy itself is not all that complicated. Getting reds and blues to work together for a purple political nation is what will be difficult.

To my colleagues and friends in red states, consider how central the care of the sick is to living with faith (pardon my very Mormon approach to this discussion of values, no offense to other faith traditions intended). And remember that high-quality health care delivered consistently to everyone is $1 trillion per year cheaper than our current system. Here is what I would like to say to you:

The prophet Ezekiel lived 2,600 years ago in the heart of what is now Iraq in the most powerful city of what was then the known world. He was a Hebrew slave laboring on the fabled Hanging Gardens of Babylon, captured during a Babylonian raid ten years before the final fall of Jerusalem and destruction of the Temple of Solomon. In a postmortem review of the causes of the downfall of the kingdom of Judah, Ezekiel said: "Woe to the shepherds of Israel who only take care of themselves! Should not the shepherds have strengthened the flock? . . .You have not strengthened the weak or healed the sick or bound up the injured" (34:2–4).

Six centuries later and only a few years before Jerusalem would again be destroyed, this time by Roman legions, another Jewish prophet spoke of the need to care for the sick. In the last parable found in the Gospel of Matthew, Christ made the point that righteous people seek out the needy to assist them, including care for the ill. "I was sick, and ye visited me," he said, and he meant all sick people, even "the least of these" (Matthew 25:36).

These words have inspired generations of Christian doctors and nurses and induced the donations that have led to the construction of many hospitals, including most of the hospitals in Utah. King Benjamin, an American Christian monarch living more than a century before Christ, made the same point: "For the sake of retaining a remission of your sins from day to day.... I would that ye should ... [visit] the sick and [administer] to their relief" (Mosiah 4:26). King Benjamin also made it clear that the care of the sick must be done wisely, which I take to mean efficiently or in a sustainable fashion. The care of the sick must be a priority for all who would follow Christ.

Americans have generally tried to live up to that Christian principle. We've built thousands of hospitals with charitable donations and taxes. Medical and nursing education has been publicly subsidized, as is most meaningful medical research. When private-sector funding for indigent and elderly medical care failed, we shouldered the dual burdens of Medicaid and Medicare. And then there are the countless other programs for the care of the sick: the Indian Health Service; the VA medical centers; the Child Health Insurance Program; Ryan White funds; family planning grants; the Women, Infants, and Children program; Children with Special Health Needs; Newborn Screening; and many others. And polling data over the years reflects our intent that every American should be able to receive the gift of health care. The Harris organization and the *Washington Post/ABC News* both found that four in five Americans support publicly funded health care for all.[18] The goodwill and generosity of the American people speak volumes about our intent. We've believed the ancient Jewish prophets: health care is a gift we want to give ourselves.

To my colleagues and friends in the blue states, consider how central the care of the sick is to living with science, public policy, and poetry. And remember that mental health services, drug and alcohol addiction treatment, services for AIDS and other STD patients, mammography and other cancer-screening services, vaccines, and a litany of other worthy health-care interventions are ultimately unaffordable when not delivered uniformly of high quality and without the administrative waste of health insurance. To you I would say:

Dr. John Symynges was one of London's most successful physicians in the late sixteenth century. He housed his family in upscale Cheapside, on Trinity Lane. He was wealthy, holding property in three counties, and widely respected throughout town. He was a senior member of the Royal Academy of Medicine. It's said he owed all of this to his shrewd business sense. His mantra for his medical practice was simple: "Before you meddle with [a patient] make your bargaine wisely now he is in paine."[19]

Quite simply, he urged fledgling doctors to settle the fee for treatment while the patient was unable to really negotiate.

Dr. Symynges and his self-serving style of practicing the business of medicine, despite his preeminence during his own lifetime, would be entirely forgotten to us now, and deservedly so, but for the accident of history that by marriage he became the stepfather of John Donne, one of England's greatest poets. John Donne received training in the law and later in life took holy orders and became the dean of St. Paul's, where he served for the last decade of his life. By this time, Donne had already become more famous than his stepfather because of the poetry he had written. However, the sermons and meditations he penned while a clergyman sealed his enduring fame. Once, while too ill to arise from his bed, he heard the church bell tolling and wrote his seventeenth meditation:

> Perchance he for whom this bell tolls may be so ill, as that he knows not it tolls for him; and perchance I may think myself so much better than I am, as that they who are about me, and see my state, may have caused it to toll for me, and I know not that. . . . The bell doth toll for him that thinks it doth. . . . No man is an

island, entire of itself; every man is a piece of the continent, a part of the main. If a clod be washed away by the sea, Europe is the less, as well as if a promontory were, as well as if a manor of thy friend's or of thine own were: any man's death diminishes me, because I am involved in mankind, and therefore never send to know for whom the bell tolls; it tolls for thee. . . . Another man may be sick, too, and sick to death, and this affliction may lie in his bowels, as gold in a mine, and be of no use to him; but this bell, that tells me of his affliction, digs out and applies that gold to me, if by this consideration of another's danger I take mine own into contemplation.[20]

Here we have an entirely different approach to the possibilities that contact with illness provides than that of the opportunistic practitioner. For Donne, illness in another, no matter how remote our contact, was to be shared, contemplated, and learned from.

Wealth generated from the sick comes not as coin but as shared human experience, for which the observer can be grateful. Applied to my professional life in clinical care, Donne's words signal me to accept my calling as a requirement to subsume my self-interest and seek to attach myself to a cause greater than my own because I am involved in mankind. Donne would have all of us contemplate our own personal danger as we make ourselves aware of the afflictions of others.

These lessons of three hundred years ago need relearning now. Medicine, once again, has been reduced to a business opportunity. In a nation where tens of millions have no financing for basic health-care services, leading to tens of thousands of preventable deaths annually, our body politic has become paralyzed by a market-oriented health policy. Bells are tolling, yet we pretend we're not diminished by the suffering of our fellow countrymen. We pretend the afflictions of the uninsured are not ours to share, as if we individually are an island entirely of itself—and this despite the fact that we pay twice as much per capita for health care than do the citizens of the rest of the developed world, mostly in the form of the highest per-person taxes for health care in the world. What we are missing is the contemplation of our own danger.

Americans are least likely in the developed world to avoid death amenable to health care. We've allowed the business of medicine to so deviate our health system from its principle mission that preventable injury to hospitalized patients has become, as mentioned in chapter 1, the fifth leading cause of death in our country.

More than ten years ago, Tony Snow, who died from colon cancer while serving the Bush White House as press secretary, made this statement: "In the real world, people stampede when somebody slaps up a sign that reads 'Free'. This is the theory behind bargain basements, but it also applies to hip replacements and appendectomies."[21]

This is Dr. Symynges's approach to medicine reiterated in modern parlance, and it makes no more sense now than it did then. I've never met a patient willing to have his appendix removed because a hospital had bargain-basement appendectomies for sale. I doubt Mr. Snow actually behaved this way when he was a patient. As far as I know, Mr. Snow did not attempt to start his course of chemotherapy before he had cancer because he found the drugs on sale. After having the experience of colon cancer, would he still maintain that Dr. Symynges's approach—to make the bargain with the patient while he is yet in pain—is the correct one? Is medicine a commodity efficiently traded and distributed by markets? Are patients shoppers or customers, or are they people for whom the bell tolls?

The *Wall Street Journal,* an authority on markets and customers, may help us with an answer. A couple of years ago, president of the National Center for Policy Analysis John C. Goodman published an opinion piece in the *WSJ* entitled "Perverse Incentives in Healthcare." The article included this thought:

> Research . . . at Dartmouth Medical School suggest[s] that if everyone in America went to the Mayo Clinic, our annual health-care bill would be 25% lower (more than $500 billion!), and the average quality of care would improve. . . .

Of course, not everyone can get treatment at Mayo. . . . But why are these examples of efficient, high quality care not being replicated all across the country? The answer is that high quality, low-cost care is not financially rewarding. Indeed, the opposite is true. Hospitals and doctors can make more money providing inefficient, mediocre care.[22]

If the statement that hospitals and doctors are paid to deliver inefficient, mediocre care confuses you, let me illustrate with data from a hospital in Central Utah. In the mid-1990s, a family physician practicing at Sanpete Community Hospital observed that patients presenting for treatment of pneumonia were not receiving optimal care and therefore were becoming sicker and dying more often than should have been the case. He organized a protocol for optimal treatment of community-acquired pneumonia, per-suaded every one of his physician colleagues at the hospital to follow it, and induced the hospital to adopt it. Almost overnight the care of pneumonia improved. Twenty-five percent fewer patients became sick enough to require hospitalization. For those patients admitted to the hospital, length of stay dropped by a third. The length of time before the instigation of proper anti-biotic treatment dropped by a quarter. And the cost per case fell by one-half.

This is the optimal outcome in a market: the quality of service goes up, and the cost drops by half. In a functioning free market, the provider of such service should be handsomely rewarded. Unfortunately for San-pete Community Hospital, there was no reward. In fact, the amount paid for pneumonia care fell even more than per-case cost; the hospital took a financial hit for providing better treatment for pneumonia. Hospitals and doctors get the best payments when they let their patients get as sick as possible. This is what Mr. Goodman meant when he said that there are perverse incentives in the American health-care system. In American health-care's business as usual, if you really want to make money caring for people with pneumonia, let them become sick enough to require inten-sive care because that is how you can make the most profitable health-care sales. The fact that American health care pays doctors to harm patients through mediocre care is evidence that market principles are not at work in health care. A market does not have perverse incentives. And a market commodity does not have a lower price for higher quality. Health care is not a commodity. Dr. Symynges was wrong. The best bargains are not driven by the patient's pain.

If you want further evidence that health care is not a market commodity, consider this: nearly $2 trillion of our nation's $3 trillion health economy comes from our taxes. What market is 60 percent tax funded? Why do we taxpayers agree to fund health care with so much tax money? Because in our hearts and minds, we know John Donne is right—any man's death diminishes me. It matters to all of us whether the uninsured tuberculosis patient receives appropriate care; his illness places society at risk. In health care, we're not supposed to believe in caveat emptor because the buyer is a patient, neither prepared nor able to shop. We place ethical obligations on physicians to serve their patients' needs ahead of their own personal interests. John Donne was right: when it comes to health care, Americans have always known that no man is an island.

Let us, both blue and red, therefore agree that health care is not a commodity that can be efficiently distributed by a market. A market exists when a completely informed buyer can freely choose to enter into a transaction with a self-interested seller without any positive externality. Market efficiency is demonstrated when demand rises as price declines. None of these conditions exist within the health-care sector.

In summary, let the formation of the purple political nation begin with recognition of the reasons why health care is not a commodity to be distributed by market forces:

a. Buyers of health care lack clinical knowledge (no caveat emptor) and are not free to decide whether to purchase health services (especially in urgent settings).

b. Sellers of health services are not supposed to act in their own self-interest, which is why society does not tolerate physicians and nurses whose greed preempts the best interests of their patients.

c. Positive externality refers to a situation when someone other than the buyer or seller has a legitimate interest in the outcome of a transaction, such as is the case when the general public has an interest in assuring the best care for a patient with a communicable disease. We have massive infusions of tax dollars into health systems because of positive externalities.

d. The inverse relationship between price and demand does not hold for health services. No one ever bought an appendectomy because it was on sale. Demand for health services is determined by epidemiology (the frequency of disease and injury), not by price.

Lack of accountability to patients in our health system is not a market failure, since health care is not a commodity efficiently distributed by market forces. Rather, lack of accountability in health systems is a social failure. For instance, preventable hospital injuries can be discovered and eliminated not by individual buyers (patients) but by public-health agencies. The pretense of markets, so characteristic of American health policy, has created perverse incentives to deliver mediocre care in an inefficient manner.[23] Reducing poor quality and inefficiency waste will require inventing new social mechanisms to replace the failing business models that characterize the American health-care delivery system.

Recently passed federal and state health "reform" legislation (the Affordable Care Act and its predecessor in Massachusetts) are coverage initiatives and not the needed reform measures. Massachusetts officials testified before Congress one year before the passage of the Affordable Care Act that burgeoning costs made the Bay State's health "reforms" financially unsustainable. Recent projections by the Congressional Budget Office confirm that the Affordable Care Act will not prevent future "excess cost growth" in health care.[24]

In summary, growth in US health-care costs far exceeds any international comparison. Coverage initiatives, the standard American health-policy approach over the past fifty years, ultimately fail to contain excessive growth in health-care costs. The business model of private health insurance is administratively wasteful and invokes perverse incentives to deliver mediocre care. Sustainable health-system reform must introduce social accountability into health-care delivery while targeting improved quality and efficiency.

One value or fact about which both reds and blues appear to agree is the value of allowing individual states to work out their own health-care policy. The Tenth Amendment to the Constitution presupposes that powers not explicitly given to the national government remain with state governments. I presume this is the explanation for why a federal public-health agency like the Centers for Disease Control does not enter into a state to begin a public-health investigation unless invited to do so by the lead state health official. Conservative politicians have long recognized that this federalism principle applies to health-care policy. For instance, while campaigning for his first term in the United States Senate, Senator Mike Lee (R-UT) stated in a televised debate (in answer to a question I posed to him as a member of the studio audience) that each state should be allowed to fashion its own policy for health-system reform, even if it meant the state would create a single-payer system. He promised to vote for any federal legislation that created the necessary law and budgetary regulations so that state-based health policy would become the rule in the United States.

The Patient Protection and Affordable Care Act contains a provision (section 1332) that anticipates exactly this kind of state-based health policy. Representative Jim McDermott (D-WA, now retired) introduced legislation (the State-Based Universal Health Care Act of 2015) that would have strengthened this provision and anticipated that states desiring something better than the health policy provided under Obamacare might seek such improvement by applying to the federal government for appropriate waivers. Representative McDermott's successor, Representative Pramila Jayapal, will soon introduce a similar bill.

Finally, at the state level, legislation by ballot initiative is possible, while there is no provision for a federal referendum. Because of the public-policy vise exerted by the medical industrial complex on Congress and the various state legislatures, a breakthrough for real health-system reform may only be possible at the ballot box. Single-payer purists who support only a federal "Medicare for All" statute need to remember that twice in the past quarter century there has been a Democrat administration coupled with dual Democrat majorities in Congress and neither time found the Democrat elected leaders even so much as allowing a congressional hearing about real, sustainable health-system reform. Let's try something new and different. Give state governments a chance to open the door for a better health policy. If one state succeeds, the improvements in health-system function will convince others to follow.

Because I believe the state I know best is my current home state, Utah, I've fashioned, by way of example, a state-based proposal for comprehensive, sustainable health-system reform in Utah.

In brief, I propose to create one new government agency (the Utah Health System Commission) and rename an existing publicly owned trust fund (the Public Employee Health Plan will be called the Utah Health Cooperative) while transforming it into the sole payment source for health services needed by Utah residents. I also propose to strengthen the current passive public-health surveillance system for patient safety into a mandatory reporting system with trained staff for interventions to improve hospital performance.

The goal is to extend comprehensive, publicly financed health benefits to every Utah citizen without increasing overall cost for health care. Utah already has the lowest per capita costs for health care in the United States, probably for three reasons: a. the overall population health in Utah is excellent, with lower rates of smoking, inebriation, and social disruption (as per Dr. Victor Fuchs, cited previously); b. Utah has the youngest age population on average, with the nation's highest birth rate; and c. many Utah hospitals are part of one of the nation's best-quality hospital systems—Intermountain Healthcare.

It doesn't hurt the cause for health-system reform that wages tend to be lower in the Beehive State (the state motto is "Industry"), since health care is a labor-intensive economic sector. Overall, conditions in Utah should be ripe for an optimal try at real health-system reform, unless the fact that Utah is the reddest political state in the nation prohibits the populace from attempting to join the purple political nation.

Here are the details of my proposed plan for reform:

1. The Utah Health System Commission will have two principle tasks: a. define the clinically proven set of health benefits for every citizen in Utah; and b. efficiently adjudicate claims against any part of the health system (i.e., in a fashion similar to workers compensation, with administrative law judges and without punitive damages or juries). The commission will be given two years after passage of the enabling statute to determine what diagnostic and therapeutic interventions have been proven effective by clinical science while being the least expensive alternative. These interventions will constitute the initial Uniform Benefit for all Utah residents. The commission will have the task of continuously reviewing clinical science as it evolves to keep the Uniform Benefit updated. The commission will also organize an administrative law system similar to the system that handles claims about workplace injuries and illnesses, for the purpose of adjudicating claims against any part of the health-care system, such as malpractice by providers or failure to make payment by the Utah Health Cooperative. The principle features of this administrative law system will be that no punitive damages will be allowed and no jury trials will be conducted. The overall effort by the commission will be to reduce/eliminate clinically inappropriate care. The Uniform Benefit is intended to include only those services which are better than marginally effective. For instance, nearsightedness would be managed with corrective lenses, not LASIK surgery. The surgery would be sold on the market, of course, but paid for privately. Some interventions wouldn't be covered at all because they're not proven to work or

are, in fact, too risky. Induction of labor would be used only for limited circumstances, for instance.

Goods, devices, and services not included in the Uniform Benefit can be sold in Utah under the proposed law but will not be paid for out of the public funds for health services administered by the Utah Health Cooperative. Defensive medicine, by definition, is clinically inappropriate care because it's ordered as a means to reduce a doctor's litigation risk and not because of medical necessity. Eliminating malpractice litigation through administrative law adjudication will vastly downsize the inappropriate care that occurs through defensive medicine, without changing a patient's constitutional right to seek redress for tort injury.

2. The Utah Health Cooperative (formerly the Public Employees Health Plan) would undergo a two-year transformation from its current role of providing efficiently paid health benefits to Utah State government and other public employees. PEHP is the most efficient payer in Utah, reporting less than 4 percent overhead, while the largest four private health insurers in the state average 15 percent administrative costs. Upon passage of the enabling legislation, PEHP would be renamed the Utah Health Cooperative and would immediately begin selling health benefits to all Utahns, whether employed in the public sector or not. Medicaid, CHIP, and other publicly paid programs would be transferred to the Utah Health Cooperative as soon as practicable. Private health insurers would have two years to phase out their Utah operations. The Utah Health Cooperative would negotiate with the US Department of Health and Human Services to become the fiscal agent for Medicare in Utah, anticipating the time when Medicare beneficiaries living in the Beehive State could be phased into full participation in the program. The most important function of the Utah Health Cooperative, aside from receiving and managing all funds intended to support health services in Utah, would be to

use its monopoly clout to improve health-system function, including better use of primary care; improved distribution of public health; optimizing behavioral health services, including addiction recovery, negotiating better prices for pharmaceuticals and medical devices; and supporting continuous quality improvement system-wide.

3. Patient injury would be reduced through standard public-health surveillance and intervention. Every hospital would be required to report all cases of preventable patient injury, as defined by the public-health authority in the state of Utah. There already exists a voluntary patient-injury reporting system in Utah, so the transformation to a mandated system of reporting wouldn't be difficult. As with case reports of communicable disease, patient-injury case reports would require public-health investigation followed by recommendations for preventive interventions. Hospital performance in patient safety would become a matter of public record. Utahns will find that when the spotlight of public accountability is shined on patient injury, hospitals will make a good faith effort to provide a better environment for patients, and patient safety will dramatically improve. There will be fewer medication errors, fewer patients falling, and fewer bedsores. These same principles can and ultimately will also be applied to extended-care facilities, renal dialysis centers, and other clinical facilities.

Based on a variety of sources,[25] a rough estimate of Utah's total health expenditures for 2009 would be $15 billion. Approximately 60 percent of US health expenditures arise from public taxation,[26] or roughly $9 billion of Utah's total 2009 health spending, leaving $6 billion from private sources (out of pocket from individuals or payments from private employers not offset by tax credits). Assuming that the relative proportions of waste due to poor quality and inefficiency cited above are applicable in Utah, approximately $6 billion of health spending in Utah during 2009 was lost to the cost of inappropriate care, patient injury, failure to deliver best-practice care, and administrative overhead. Therefore, improved quality and efficiency anticipated through the proposed health-system reform would substantially reduce (essentially eliminate?) the need for health-care funds from private sources not offset by tax credits or mandated by law. The proposal accordingly anticipates that program funding will be principally derived through maintaining current public revenue streams paying for health care. There are currently three major public revenue streams: (1) publicly funded health-care programs, including Medicaid, Medicare, CHIP, IHS, and a multitude of smaller health-service programs ($4 billion); (2) assorted tax credits for employer/employee purchase of health benefits/care ($4 billion); and (3) funding for federal, state, and local government employee/retiree/dependent health care plus government mandated health-service payments for workers compensation, vehicle insurance, etc. ($2 billion). During the initial two years after passage of enabling legislation, while the Utah Health Systems Commission is organizing the Uniform Benefit, the state of Utah will be required to assure the preservation of these public revenue streams for health care by: (1) negotiating with the national government for full carryover of all federal health-care funding into a block grant to the state of Utah to be deposited with the Utah Health Cooperative; (2) identifying all state and local tax funding for health care, including budgets for purchasing health benefits for all public employees and redirecting those funds in perpetuity to the Utah Health Cooperative; and (3) organizing an equitable levy of private employers and individuals, partially offset by federal and state tax credits, equal to the current level of tax supported health benefits purchased voluntarily in the private sector or mandated by law. Employers will no longer need to purchase the health-care benefit associated with workers compensation insurance, since all illness and injury care will be funded by one source. They will also be able to substantially downsize human-resource costs since employment-based health insurance will no longer be needed. Further, the oft-cited cost shift of the un- and underinsured onto employment-based health insurance will disappear.

For all of these reasons, business in Utah will be much better with the Utah Health Cooperative taking on universal health-care financing.

State-based health-system reform is not intended to be an end run around established federal law, policy, and budgeting related to health care. Medicare is perhaps the most popular governmental program in the history of our nation, maybe challenged only by the GI benefits after World War II. American seniors have come to depend upon Medicare paying the bulk of their health-care costs during their retirement and twilight years. I myself am approaching the age of Medicare eligibility, and in no way do I intend to give up this cornerstone of my retirement planning. Rather, I intend state-based health-system reform to finish the job Congress started fifty years ago when Medicare was initially passed. Let it no longer be the case that there is a generational cost shift of health-care expenses from the elderly, who tend to have more resources, to the middle-aged and younger working-age population, who tend to be in the early aspects of asset accumulation.

Let's apply the benefit package afforded for seniors on Medicare to all Americans but allow states with the political will to make that happen do so with federal oversight and funding but state initiative and governance. States that don't, at least initially, have the political will to organize a best-practice health-care system can and will remain on Obamacare, which itself has now been tested through litigation and is the law of the land.

The first step toward meaningful state health-system reform is passage of a State-Based Universal Healthcare Act. This will of necessity be an act of Congress, though it's already anticipated in the Patient Protection and Affordable Care Act (Obamacare). The medical industrial complex is arrayed in all its formidable force against passage of any form of the State-Based Universal Healthcare Act. Congress, as currently constituted, listens to the medical industrial complex, so right now, as I write this paragraph (in 2017), there is no chance that the 115th Congress will pass this legislation. If you want to take a step toward the purple political nation we need for sustainable health-system reform, you will ask every candidate for federal office within the sound of your voice (or email, or Facebook, etc.) whether they will support the State-Based Universal Healthcare Act.

No matter what they may say to you (and they will say as little as they can get away with), don't believe the answer. Rather, check to see if the bill has been passed. If it hasn't, the next time you vote, vote every federal elected official on your ballot out of office and begin asking the next set to support the bill. Don't worry about which party will inherit the seat in Congress or the White House. Worry only about whether whoever is in office actively supports the bill. You'll have the opportunity to throw your new congressman out of office in only two years if he or she likewise fails to get the job done. We can only care about results in the purple political nation, not party affiliation.

I guarantee you that if federal elected officials find themselves unelected because of failure to pass the State-Based Universal Healthcare Act, eventually Congress will pass the bill.

Whatever form state-based health-system reform takes, assuming we Americans can make it happen in at least one state in a purple political nation, we will need a way of recognizing that sustainable reform has occurred, because we can't trust the political class to tell us anything other than what they think we want to hear. How will the Simon family know that their elected leaders are succeeding in real health-system reform? First, in a sustainable health-care system, enrollment in a health-care plan will be easy, even automatic. For instance, in Utah, if my proposed plan were to become the law, all Utah residents (however the Utah Legislature chooses to define residency) would become beneficiaries of the Utah Health Cooperative. No complicated shopping (online or otherwise) would be required. Second, out-of-pocket expenses would disappear. Copayments, coinsurance, premiums, point-of-service payments, and any other patient-fleecing mechanisms ever dreamed up by the creative minds of the health-insurance bureaucracy would be eliminated. Health care would be publicly funded, as it mostly already is in the United States. We Americans have been generous with our taxes for health care; sustainable health-system reform will efficiently use those tax revenues without demanding out-of-pocket payments and without burdening future generations by deficit spending now.

Third, the Simons and every other Utah family will be able to choose their own doctors and hospitals. No worrying about who is in or out of network because the network will be all physicians and other health care professionals in the entire state willing to work with the Utah Health Cooperative. Fourth, there will be no more bake sales to raise funds for a neighbor's cancer treatment. Personal bankruptcy due to the cost of illness and injury care will not exist after the passage of sustainable health-system reform, just as is the case in every other first-world nation. Medically necessary and appropriate care will be available to all Utahns. Angela Simons will be able to use her inhaler as prescribed. Fifth, society will stop criminalizing those with mental illness and addiction. Behavioral-health services will become part of the mainstream health-care system, and needed services will be available to treat these often-chronic disorders.

The purple world as described by my infectious-disease professor, the world of microbiological exposure, does exist. By now we have become accustomed to the recurrent appearance of the latest microbial menace making news headlines worldwide: Ebola, bird flu, SARS, and AIDS have all taken a turn at being the new communicable disease-causing apprehension on a large scale. As potentially risky as the microbial world can be, however, it has never been nearly as purple (or risky to human health) as is the current approach to health-care delivery in the United States. In America, unlike any other first-world nation, tens of thousands of people die from causes that known medical science could treat, merely because they don't have the financing to pay for diagnosis and/or treatment.

What's worse, these people who are unnecessarily dying are taxpayers or dependents of taxpayers who pay the highest taxes for health care in the world. Further, for those Americans who do manage to have the wherewithal to get into the health-care delivery system, the risk of health-care business as usual becomes worse. Half of American patients will not receive the clinically proven care they need. Over a hundred thousand more each year will die from preventable patient injury. Many thousands of surgeries and other medical interventions will be clinically inappropriate and not have any reasonable chance to improve the health of the patient. Those are the results of the purple world of perverse incentives in American health care. Rather than being frightened by news reports of the latest microbial scourge, Americans should be purple with rage about the egregious state of affairs in our health-care system.

So, be politically purple. Rid yourself of partisan bias and begin the heavy political lifting that is the only possible remedy for the massive waste of the medical industrial complex.

Notes

1. PolitiFact-rated statements similar to this "true" when made by Senator Bernie Sanders. Please see the last chapter for complete references in support of the factual assertions in this book.

2. Wendy Moore, *The Knife Man: The Extraordinary Life and Times of John Hunter, Father of Modern Surgery* (New York: Broadway Books), 2005.

3. J. J. Ross, "The Knife Man: The Extraordinary Life and Times of John Hunter, Father of Modern Surgery," *New England Journal of Medicine* (December 1, 2005): 353, 2412–13.

4. "Washington Is Obsolete," *The Washington Post* (October 15, 2005): 353, 2412–13, https://www.washingtonpost.com/opinions/washington-is-obsolete/2015/10/15/cb3bbf8c-7109-11e5-8248-98e0f5a2e830_story.html?utm_term=.cbbab853c2c3.

5. Victor R. Fuchs, *Who Shall Live* (New York: Basic Books, 1974), 52–54.

6. "Free Market Ideology Doesn't Work for Health Care," June 8, 2015, The Center for Public Integrity, https://www.publicintegrity.org/2015/06/08/17460/free-market-ideology-doesnt-work-health-care.

7. *American Journal of Public Health* 80, no. 2 (February 1990): 209–10.

8. *Western Journal of Medicine* 154, no. 1 (January 1991): 40–42.

9. "Dr. Carl J. Johnson—Star Witness for Radiation Hysteria," February 7, 2012, http://www.falloutradiation.com/files/StarWitnessForRadiationHysteria.pdf

10. "Cobalt Cardiomyopathy: A Report of Two Cases from Mineral Assay Laboratories and a Review of the Literature," *Journal of Occupational Medicine* 34, no. 6 (June 1992): 620–26.

11. In Catalog of Arts and Artifacts, Massachusetts General Hospital, catalog no. 119 (2013), http://history.massgeneral.org/catalog/Detail.aspx?itemId=119&searchFor=churchill.

12. See J. Q. Jarvis and P. R. Morey, "Allergic respiratory disease and extraordinary microbial remediation in a building in a subtropical climate," *Applied Occupational and Environmental Hygiene* 16, no. 3 (2001): 380–88.

13. "Americans Are Getting Gored on Horns of Health-Care Dilemma," *Deseret News,* December 10, 2000, https://www.deseretnews.com/article/797312/Americans-are-getting-gored-on-horns-of-health-care-dilemma.html.

14. "Wrong Prescription? The Failed Promise of the Affordable Care Act," July 2015, https://harpers.org/archive/2015/07/wrong-prescription/, 1–2.

15. Ibid., 4.

16. Ibid., 10.

17. See "Up With Extremism," *New York Times,* January 6, 2016, https://mobile.nytimes.com/2016/01/06/opinion/up-with-extremism.html.

18. The Harris Poll, 1998; *Washington Post/ABC News,* 2003.

19. In John Stubbs, *John Donne, the Reformed Soul: A Biography* (New York: W. W. Norton, 2006), 42.

20. *The Broadview Anthology of English Literature, Volume 2: The Renaissance and the Early Seventeenth Century,* 3d ed., ed. Joseph Black and others (Ontario, Canada: Broadview Press, 2016), 835.

21. Exibit C: Silver Document, Nevada Legislature slideshow (March 4, 2004), https://www.leg.state.nv.us/Session/72nd2003/Interim/NonLeg/Silver/exhibits/11644C.pdf.

22. "Perverse Incentives in Health Care (April 5, 2007), https://www.wsj.com/articles/SB117573825899360526.

23. Ibid.

24. Congressional Budget Office, "Reducing the Deficit: Spending and Revenue Options," March 2011.

25. Kaiser State Health Facts; NCSL; Medical Expenditure Panel Survey; NME data, etc.

26. Woolhandler, *Health Affairs* 21, no. 4 (2002): 88.

About the Author

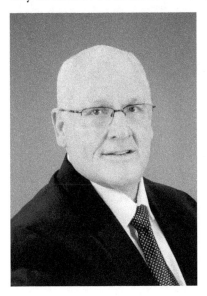

J OSEPH Q. JARVIS MD, MSPH, received his medical and public-health training at the University of Utah. He practiced family medicine in low-income clinics in Salt Lake City and Reno. He has been on the faculty of schools of medicine in Utah, Nevada, and Colorado. Dr. Jarvis was a public-health official at the US Department of Labor, the Nevada Division of Health, and the Colorado Department of Public Health and Environment. For the past twenty years, Dr. Jarvis has been a public and environmental health consultant to clients from Guam to New York City. He currently resides in Salt Lake City, Utah, with his wife, Annette, who is a corporate bankruptcy attorney. Together they have five children and seven grandchildren.

Note to the Reader

THANK YOU so much for taking the time to read *The Purple World*. I hope you are shocked to learn about the harm done by the business model of American health care. Let your outrage motivate you to act—find a way to become a force of reckoning.

If you found this message impactful, it would mean a great deal to me if you'd leave me a review on Amazon and Goodreads—and, even more, if you'd get out in the next election and vote in a way that will revitalize health care. The patient must become the priority, not the almighty dollar. Please spread the word so that others will find this book and we can gain support!

With deepest gratitude,
Dr. Joseph Q. Jarvis

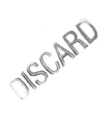

CPSIA information can be obtained
at www.ICGtesting.com
Printed in the USA
LVHW041529231219
641484LV00005B/989/P

9 780998 625485